1 on or before
below

TRY

OXFORD MEDICAL PUBLICATIONS

The Making of a Doctor

The Making of a Doctor
Medical Education in Theory and Practice

R. S. DOWNIE

Professor of Moral Philosophy
University of Glasgow

and

BRUCE CHARLTON

Lecturer in Anatomy
University of Glasgow

With chapters contributed by

K. C. CALMAN

Chief Medical Officer

and

JAMES McCORMICK

Emeritus Professor of Community Health
Trinity College, Dublin

Oxford   New York   Tokyo
OXFORD UNIVERSITY PRESS
1992

Oxford University Press, Walton Street, Oxford OX2 6DP
Oxford New York Toronto
Delhi Bombay Calcutta Madras Karachi
Petaling Jaya Singapore Hong Kong Tokyo
Nairobi Dar es Salaam Cape Town
Melbourne Auckland
and associated companies in
Berlin Ibadan

Oxford is a trade mark of Oxford University Press

Published in the United States
by Oxford University Press, New York

A catalogue record for this book is available from the British Library

Library of Congress Cataloging in Publication Data
Downie, R. S. (Robert Silcock)
The making of a doctor: medical education in theory and practice
/ R. S. Downie, Bruce Charlton; with chapters contributed
by K. C. Calman and James McCormick.
(Oxford medical publications)
Includes bibliographical references and index.
1. Medical education. I. Charlton, Bruce. II. Title. III. Series.
[DNLM: 1. Education, Medical. W 18 D751m]
R735.D69 1992 610'.71'1—dc20 92–13057

ISBN 0–19–262136–X

Set in 10.5/12pt Palatino
by Graphicraft Typesetters Ltd., Hong Kong
Printed in Great Britain by Biddles Ltd., Guildford & King's Lynn

Foreword
Professor D. A. Shaw

Today's medical education, its style and content, are major determinants of the quality of tomorrow's health services. Medical education excites discussion, much of it critical, not only within the profession but also in the wider public forum. In recent years interest has been heightened both by developments in educational theory and practice and also by changes in the organization of health care systems. Contributions to the debate, especially those that are original and provocative, are timely and welcome.

Most systems that have a capacity for change are subject to conflicting interests. Undergraduate medical education is under constant pressure to extend its scope to encompass the ever-increasing knowledge and technology that attach to existing disciplines, and that in some cases create new ones hitherto unrepresented in the curriculum; at the same time, it is under pressure to reduce the oppressive burden of information that it currently inflicts on our students. Medical educators are urged to adopt teaching and learning methods that demand additional resources while being beleaguered by fiscal constraints. The educators are susceptible to the allure of fresh ideas and new discoveries, but conscious of their obligation to existing service needs. They recognize that the medical school organization that is ideal for educational purposes may conflict with the perceived interests of departments or their individual members in relation to research or career development. They also recognize that many dilemmas facing the practising profession, such as the balance between the demands of individuals and of populations, or the ethics of prioritization, must needs be reflected in the process of education.

The challenge to medical education must be to reconcile these tensions and to find a *via media* that balances the many and varied demands that are placed upon it. There is almost universal agreement about one area in which a degree of imbalance is in need of urgent correction. The explosive growth of knowledge in medicine and its related sciences has resulted in an intolerable degree of overcrowding of the undergraduate curriculum. Our students are so overwhelmed by the burden of facts that intellectual stimulation is lost, critical faculties are under-developed, and curiosity is dimmed. There is a consensus that the educational as opposed to the professional aims of the medical course must be revived and that a framework in which they can flourish must be established. The worry is that such good intentions have been proclaimed on a great many occasions in the past without redressing the tyranny of the information overload. The fulfilment of the intentions will require changes in organization that go beyond the details of the curriculum, and changes in approaches and attitudes to learning that will enable doctors to adapt to advances in knowledge and technology throughout their professional lives.

These challenges are admirably addressed in the chapters of this book of which the 'author-mix' ensures originality of approach and scholarly exploration of the dimensions of learning and of doctoring. Inevitably there will be those who dissent from some of the views expressed, or reject their harsher strictures. But all who are concerned about the future of medical education will be stimulated by the analysis of the problems and the suggestions for their solution. The medical profession enjoys the unique privilege of determining how our doctors should be educated. Responsibility for implementing changes that are necessary for the long term benefit of society rests with us.

Preface

Medical education, like all aspects of education, is under intense scrutiny from the government and the general public. The government requires doctors to be financially accountable, and the general public wishes them to be wise and humane as well as technically competent. We argue that all of these goals can be achieved without increased expenditure, but cannot be achieved merely by tinkering with the present system. Too often the discussion of medical education is a matter for consenting medical professors in private and largely consists of carving up the curriculum to satisfy the demands of various academic departments. This does not make for educational progress.

The book takes a broad perspective in order to examine the moral, philosophical, and historical underpinnings of medical education. Our suggestions for change are inevitably radical, but nevertheless they are firmly rooted in the excellences of existing medical education — and we find much to admire in the present system. Moreover, the changes we recommend need not be implemented all at once; we are gradualists rather than revolutionaries and our concern is with a lifetime of medicine — from selection for medical school until retirement from practice. Our overriding objective throughout is to suggest that it is both desirable and possible to put *education* back into medical training.

We wish to give grateful acknowledgment for the help and encouragement we have received from others. Professor David Shaw has wide experience of the problems of medical education from his time as Professor of Neurology and Dean of Medicine at Newcastle and, more recently, as Chairman of the Education Division of the General Medical Council. He has kindly contributed a foreword; it should be emphasized that the views expressed therein are his own. Dr Kenneth Calman, Chief Medical Officer and formerly Professor of Postgraduate Medical Education, has written chapters on the pre-registration year and on continuing medical education, and has allowed us to draw on previous collaborative work. Professor James McCormick of Trinity College, Dublin, has contributed a chapter on general practice, another area where specialist knowledge is essential. Dr Johanna Geyer-Kordesch and Dr Marguerite Dupree of the Wellcome Unit for the History of Medicine at Glasgow have discussed some historical points with us, and Elizabeth Telfer of the Department of Philosophy has discussed philosophical points and allowed us to draw on previous collaborative work. Since medical education is a broad area the book could not have been written without the help and encouragement of these colleagues. But responsibility for the views expressed, apart from the contributed chapters, remains with us. Finally, we acknowledge prompt, efficient, and patient assistance from our secretaries, Anne Valentine and Anne Southall.

Glasgow   R. S. D.
December 1991   B. C.

Contents

PART III: CHALLENGES

1 Introduction: stating the problem

Why write a book about medical education? The simplest answer is that medical education is important and should be done well. But is it being done well?

It is our belief that medical education is flawed in several important respects. Furthermore, we believe that useful things can be done to improve the situation. The 1970s saw a debate on the subject which was international in its scope and radical in its conclusions; many criticisms were made, and many solutions were proposed. However, at the end of the day we find the state of medical education is qualitatively very similar to its state before the talking began — although the quantity and balance have altered in several respects.

The problem with many earlier discussions of medical education was that they were utopian. They took as their starting-point a blank slate upon which they could write their curricula, and a blank cheque with which to employ new staff using new methods and build brand-new integrated medical colleges. They did not take account of the implications for resources: the problems of running a clinical service parallel to the needs for teaching, and the requirement for research as well as teaching within a university setting. There was also a tendency to confine discussion to the undergraduate curriculum, whereas medical education begins with selection into medical school and ends only when the doctor retires from practice.

In this book we take as our starting-point the place we are at just now: the people, the methods, the buildings, the funding. This is clearly variable between different medical schools and different regions and in different specialties. Having found out just where we are, and why, we are then in a position to work from this towards improvements. In terms of a political analogy, this approach is known as gradualism or permeation: it is the method advocated by the liberal democratic wing of the Labour Party or the traditionalist style of Conservatism, as opposed to the hard-liners on either side. In most situations it is not necessary to construct a complete blueprint for utopia.

We do not need to know exactly where we are going in order to set off in the right direction. Moreover, it is not necessary to know in advance the exact point at which change should stop; this is more easily decided when the practical consequences become apparent rather than predicted on theoretical grounds. On the other hand, it may be helpful to suggest what need *not* be included in medical education. There is a temptation to include in the ideal medical education every factor which makes for health and well-being. This must be resisted as unrealistic. Doctors are only one of several professional groups aiming at health and well-being.

Our analysis of medicine in the narrow sense nevertheless aims to be comprehensive: from admission as a student to retirement. The problems and consequences of education can be appreciated by observing the dilemmas of imaginary students and doctors in a variety of possible situations. These we describe in the 'vignettes' which introduce many of the chapters. Medical education can be regarded as a system of evolving goals and frameworks throughout the working life of a practising doctor; a continuing process, with different problems and priorities at each stage.

What happens during medical education? The answers are far from straightforward, and depend on the perspective from which medicine is viewed. To the outsider medical training looks very much like a process of indoctrination — or pro-fessionalization, to give it a more polite title. To the social scien-tist, the sheer length of the training stems from the need to establish standards of conformity to the group. It is often said that what follows is a progressive desensitization to the patient's point of view. To combat this, medicine must be seen in relation to the rest of society, because the role of medicine is partially determined by forces operating from outside the profession. This in turn should influence the way that doctors are trained.

If random samples of doctors were asked about the problems of medical education it is likely that they would concentrate on the problems of teaching clinical skills to students and junior doctors. Such questions as the nature of examinations might also be raised, as might the balance and relevance of the various curricula. These are all topics of great importance; but the process of medical education is much wider than this, and these problems are probably not the most significant in terms of outcome.

There is a tendency for medical education to be a 'top-down' process, where those at the summit of the profession dictate to the broad base of educators. But medical education is of wider interest than this. A large range of teachers and experts are involved in the training of doctors, and the public will also have strong views. Furthermore, the pressures upon specialist doctors may tend to produce a distorted picture of medicine as a whole, and the temptation to pursue a 'hidden agenda' of building up their own specialty at the expense of the broad picture. From our position as relative 'outsiders' to the world of medicine we hope to avoid these pitfalls: to take an overview of the subject, with different points given their due weight.

There is of course an academic specialty of medical education, from which we have learned a great deal. But our view is that it is important at this time of change to involve many others in the debate, both medical and non-medical. For this reason we have avoided detailed academic references, which tend to confine the debate to positions familiar only to 'insiders', and have provided only a few highly selective suggestions for further reading. We try to be both philosophical and pragmatic, both radical and practical.

The attitude to the whole subject of medical education among doctors is usually negative. Those who are interested in it are often regarded as second-rate and boring. The periods when 'education' is important are seen as something to be got through as painlessly as possible before the real business of practising medicine can begin. In a sense this is a healthy attitude — at any given time most effort should go into doing rather than thinking about doing. However, in some hospital specialties the 'getting-through' can actually take longer than the practising life of a typical consultant; for example in some branches of surgery. So 'training mania' represents one powerful trend in medical practice. If training is going to take up such vast quantities of time and resources, it is vital that we check to see if it is necessary and effective.

All too often there is no attempt to justify the nature of medical education beyond an exhortation from those further up the ladder to 'trust us, we know what we are doing'. The various hurdles can all too easily become ends in themselves, detached entirely from any conception of what they are supposed to be for. This is exemplified by the peculiarly British hobby of collecting letters to put after one's name. A strange state may result in which students or junior doctors 'forget' where they are going — that the *real* job is either to be a consultant or a principal GP — and instead regard this as a kind of *reward* for being a good junior — a time to relax and/or make a bit of money.

So, although the education of medical students and junior doctors will concern us for much of this book, we will not neglect the fact that most of medicine is, or should be, done by consultants and GPs, who will usually be in the job for periods in excess of thirty years. Given the changes in practice over the last thirty years it is foolish to assume that principals — no matter how well trained and rigorously examined — can coast along on the knowledge and skills they learned two decades ago. Continuing Medical Education (CME) is thus seen not as a luxury, an optional extra, but as the key to good medical practice.

On the other hand, isolating a key area is not the same thing as taking effective action. For example, the vital importance of CME does not mean that *anything* can count as satisfactory. In a world of limited time and money it is essential to evaluate whether or not your cherished schemes are, at the end of the day, having the intended effect. And if they are not having any useful effect, then they should be abandoned without regret, and something else be given a chance.

We are concerned with practical change. This means that we are interested in change where it is most needed and where it can be implemented without the requirement for massive in-jections of funding. The days of an expanding system are over; if we require money to expand one activity, then it has to come from cuts in something else. Our suggestions for change will therefore be focused on those areas where it can do the most good. There is no sense in trying to change everything at once.

So, although our discussion and analysis will cover the whole of medical education in order to see how it fits together, its strengths and weaknesses, our strategies for change will be focused and specific. Some areas of the process will be seen to be as near to perfection as we can reasonably expect, in an imperfect world and given the varied aptitudes of the individuals concerned; these, we will put aside. But other parts leave a great deal to be desired, and it is upon these latter parts that we shall concentrate.

With this in mind, we have asked two distinguished experts to contribute chapters on specific areas of current concern. Dr Calman writes of the special problems of the pre-registration year and the vital subject of CME. Professor McCormick presents a view of medical education from the viewpoint of general practice, which many commentators consider to be the most exciting direction for medical education in the future.

We live at a time of growing debate concerning the role of the doctor. There is a measure of agreement on the problems, but the solutions have become highly polarized. Two extreme opposite goals are prevalent: the 'holistic doctor', who treats the whole patient for every dysfunction and affliction of a physical, psychological, or moral nature; or the humble 'shop-keeper', who minds his or her own business, treats the specific complaints, and leaves the patient with the maximum autonomy (medicine as a consumer-driven service). Both views are radical, and both have implications for medical education. Whatever the future holds, it seems likely that the stern but kindly, condescending paternalism of the fictional Doctor Cameron is not going to survive much longer — the public is demanding more respect from its doctors; and the Government is demanding that doctors submit to external scrutiny.

It is impossible to give a satisfactory answer to the perennial question: 'What makes a good doctor?' There are surely a number of answers, and much depends on the circumstances of the health service and the society in which the doctor practises. For such reasons, it is hard to be sure that the changes we propose will make better doctors. Equally, it is clear that complacency can result only in declining standards. We can, however, be confident of the need to put *education* back into medical training. Generally speaking, we feel that if the parts are properly educational the whole will take care of itself. There will always, of course, be a place in medical practice for the expert technician — but only in the context of a broadly educated medical profession.

Part I: Theory

2 Gentlemen, tradesmen, and technicians: a brief history of medical education

The outsider coming to look at medical education might be puzzled as to why things are at present done the way they are. Although these questions are usually answered by reference to rational present-day educational criteria — what is needed — in reality the answers are as often as not related to the vicissitudes of the history of medicine. In other words, present-day education can be a matter of what happens to have *survived*, rather than what is needed.

Medical education is a part of the history of medicine, and it emerged as a subject which we could begin to discuss at the same time as medicine became a more-or-less unified profession. Indeed, medical education was itself one major defining feature of the unification of medicine: a doctor is a person who, by necessity, has passed through specific stages of medical education. So the history of medical education is intimately entwined with the history of medical practice; but once they had been established and discriminated the one from the other, the educational side began to interact with the practical side of the subject, in ways which have sometimes been beneficial, and at other times harmful.

2.1 Key stages

Modern historical opinion regards it as a mistake to describe medical education as having been propelled by the major acts of medical legislation. On the contrary, it is more accurate to regard the major items of parliamentary legislation as having simply recognized and validated states of affairs which were already established. This applies in particular to the Apothecaries Act of 1815, but also to the Medical Act of 1858 and its Amendment Act of 1886.

Historically, there was no single, defined pathway by which a 'doctor' was trained, certificated, and regulated; there was no consensus of even the broadest kind about which were the appropriate skills and knowledge for a person whose job was to deal with sick people. Indeed, up until the late eighteenth and early nineteenth centuries there were several reputable healers who undertook this role as a sideline to their main profession (which might be that of a priest, or simply a gentleman of independent means). And of course the unlearned leeches (or, less generously, 'quacks' — a name derived either from the practice of 'quacking' their wares in the marketplace, or from the 'quacksalber' or mercury frequently used as a treatment for venereal diseases) were vastly more numerous, and more respectable, in a situation where there was no recognized system of preparation or licensing for practice.

A present-day analogue to eighteenth-century medicine would be the situation prevailing in psychotherapy. Psychotherapy is offered by psychiatrists, as its highest-status (and best-paid) practitioners (equivalent, in this sense, to the physicians); but also by psychologists, social workers, health visitors and other nurses, probation officers, and several other professions. It is also offered by lay therapists, who may either subscribe to some existing school of therapy (Jungian, *Gestalt*, Reichian, or whatever) or perhaps use a system of their own invention (such as the various holistic, alternative, or 'green' mystics and priests/priestesses) — some of these being untrained and unregistered. However, while there is a fairly clear scale of prestige, the unlicensed ('quack') therapists are not regarded by the public as necessarily wicked or unethical; many people would use their services in certain situations — and this is more-or-less equivalent to the eighteenth-century attitude to medicine as a whole.

Broadly speaking, the present-day doctor evolved from a tripartite division of medicine into physicians, surgeons, and apothecaries. At the time when the medical profession began to crystallize into its present form (about the middle of the eighteenth century) the three groups were entirely independent in their organization, but overlapped very substantially in their practice. Any comments about them are therefore necessarily generalizations.

Physicians were the gentlemen healers. They were therefore educated in the 'liberal arts', such as the classics, mathematics, and (especially in Scotland) philosophy — that is to say theoretically rather than practically educated. Physicians might therefore be expected to have attended university and to hold an MA degree — although in fact graduation was the exception rather than the rule. In addition they might have obtained an MD degree, which was awarded on the basis of studying the medical authors of antiquity (Oxford and Cambridge), or a relatively highly structured course of lectures on medical topics (Edinburgh, Glasgow, and some of the continental medical schools); or the degree might have been 'bought' on the basis of established medical practice together with written testimonials (St Andrew's and Aberdeen).

Physicians were thus most closely connected with the universities. However, there was also an alternative route by which a licence to practise physic might be obtained from the corporations of physicians: the various colleges of London, Edinburgh, Glasgow, or Dublin. Perhaps their major role was in protecting the financial interests of their members by attempting, without much success, to enforce their monopolies. In this and other ways the corporations were descendants of the medieval guilds. As are the Colleges today, they were almost entirely examining, rather than teaching, bodies.

The physician was concerned with internal medicine. Aside from feeling the pulse, and observing the urine and faeces, practice involved history-taking, elaborate diagnosis based on theoretical pathology and considered opinion, and specific prescribing (in other words, a similar process to present-day homoeopathic medicine, although based on a different system). What physicians did not do was as important as what they did — they did not examine, they did not operate, they did not dispense medicine.

History-taking was detailed, but might be done at second hand; by letter or through the apothecary. The physician was therefore defined positively by status (a gentleman), by education (theoretical — a graduate or the equivalent), and by the right to prescribe; and defined negatively, by detachment from manual labour (not touching or operating on the patient; who might, after all, be a poor person!), and by detachment from association with the tradesmanlike activities of running a pharmacy.

These two major gaps in the role of the physician — not touching and not dispensing — were filled by the surgeon and the apothecary. These healers were originally of a lower status, perhaps closer to that of a middle-class tradesman than to that of a gentleman (although this, again, was subject to exceptions). Surgeons were originally members of a guild shared with barbers (and, before that, bath-attendants!); while apothecaries were a branch of the retail grocers until the Society of Apothecaries was founded in 1615. Training of both groups was by apprenticeship — helping with the running of a shop and . gradually learning the skills of the trade. Alternatively, surgeons might have obtained their experience in the army, with its enhanced opportunities for amputation.

Surgeons began to increase their status to rival that of the physicians by breaking away from the barbers and establishing a Company of Surgeons in 1745, which became a Royal College in 1800. Their prestige was enhanced by association with the then flourishing science of anatomy. Aside from performing operations, the surgeon also had responsibility for external medicine, such as the skin (which has since become part of 'internal' medicine — as dermatology) and the eye (which has continued as part of surgery up until the present — as ophthalmology). Furthermore, there was sometimes an overlap between surgery and the activities of another type of medical practitioner, the 'man midwife' (which overlap has since developed into the semi-surgical specialty of obstetrics and gynaecology).

The apothecary was originally supposed to be simply a compounder and seller of medicines — a shopkeeper; he was not allowed to charge for attendance because this encroached on the privileges of the physician (who was not allowed to dispense). However, physicians were not widely distributed outside the large cities, and anyway charged high fees, so that apothecaries began to visit patients, make the diagnosis, decide on treatment, and then make most of their income from selling the necessary drugs. Apothecaries thus began to evolve into an early form of what we would call the general practitioner.

2.2 Evolution or revolution?

Medical education has evolved gradually, and there has never been a revolution in the sense of a rapid, wholesale, and universal change. And education evolved alongside practice, so that the most profound changes in medical education were roughly simultaneous with the arrival of 'scientific' medicine in Britain during the middle of the nineteenth century. Newman (1957) describes three systems of medical practice which have been dominant, one after the other, since about 1800. At the beginning of the century the medical (specifically, the physicianly) way of practice was as described above: long, detailed history-taking with elaborate classification of symptoms; diagnosis using a purely theoretical system of pathology; and symptomatic treatment of a frequently elaborate nature (there was a 'cure' for every conceivable ailment under this system). The role of authority, judgement, and experience were paramount. Such practice went along with the purely theoretical education, combined with some experience of 'walking the wards'. The clinical experience seems to have involved looking at cases and hearing the remarks of the physician concerning treatment; there was no deliberate instruction — it was a system of pure apprenticeship.

During the early to middle part of the nineteenth century medicine underwent a radical change; emphasis shifted from symptoms and treatment to signs and diagnosis. Physical signs and examination of the patient became the subject of greatest attention; and these signs were then correlated with pathological changes following death. Diagnosis was therefore ultimately based on physical (pathological) change. Treatment was to be applied scientifically, and directed at curing the underlying physical abnormalities which caused the disease. The educational corollary was that medical education (and examination) was primarily concerned with elucidation of physical signs for the purpose of diagnosis. This included use of the stethoscope (introduced in 1819). Newman emphasizes that auscultation thus came *before* inspection, palpation, or percussion — doctors hardly examined patients before the middle of the nineteenth century. The clinician was thenceforth admired

mainly for skill in eliciting objective physical signs and applying simple, rational diagnostic schemes and treatments; and for
knowledge of pathology.

The science of correlating signs with pathology was gradually refined, without being qualitatively transformed, by technical improvements in instruments (better stethoscopes, and then
tendon hammers and later auriscopes and ophthalmoscopes;
and improved microscopes in pathology). However, during the
twentieth century there has been a further profound shift,
towards laboratory sciences as the most fundamental basics for
medicine. In present-day practice the laboratory findings carry
the greatest weight, and therapy is principally directed towards
the correction of laboratory-defined abnormalities. Thus microbiology, haematology, biochemistry, imaging, and many other
sciences are the mainstay of diagnosis and treatment (and even
when they are not available, for example in general practice,
they are used implicitly to validate interventions). The rise of
laboratory medicine has had far-reaching influences on the
content of medical education, although not perhaps as far-
reaching as it should have had.

We can see that although Newman's description of practice
is broadly true, the prevailing medical system is always heavily influenced by what went before. In particular, medical
education always seems to have been deeply nostalgic —
instead of educating for the future it hankers for the past. So the
present undergraduate curriculum retains a strong interest in
elaborate and systematic history-taking (despite its often being
impossible in everyday clinical practice), and an even stronger
emphasis on eliciting physical signs (even when these have
been proved to be useless): while the rational interpretation and
use of laboratory data are virtually ignored, or at best left to be
absorbed by osmosis.

The system of medicine has evolved slowly, therefore, drag-
ging medical education — kicking and screaming — behind it.
So much for the content. As for the form of education, this has
changed equally profoundly, although once again gradually
and in a piecemeal fashion. It is worth remembering that even
today there are three methods of licensing for medical practice
— by university degree, by conjoint or triple qualifications from
the various Royal Colleges of physicians and surgeons, and

licence from the Society of Apothecaries — although the universities overwhelmingly dominate the system, both in terms of quantity of graduates, and because they actually train the British medical students who subsequently take the licentiate exams. But in the nineteenth century licences from the various corporations were the normal qualifications.

Furthermore, both universities and corporations were primarily examining bodies, and a prescribed course of study and place of residence were seldom required. Students could prepare for their examinations by various combinations of apprenticeship with a registered practitioner; 'walking the wards' of 'teaching' hospitals; and attendance at courses of lectures given by a range of institutions, which included the universities and (to a lesser extent) the medical corporations, but also extra-mural private colleges attended part-time (early morning and late evening). These private colleges were sometimes of great eminence (perhaps the eighteenth-century anatomy schools of William and John Hunter are the best known). This peripatetic mode of study was named *lernfreiheit*, and was applied widely throughout Europe, reaching its highest development in Germany. But by the end of the nineteenth century the medical training was much more unified in time and place, with a standardized full-time curriculum based in a single university or teaching hospital: the extra-mural colleges gradually lost prestige and popularity, and died out completely some time before the foundation of the NHS.

Another major change was the evolution of the general practitioner. At the beginning of the nineteenth century the medical profession was divided into the 'three estates' of physicians, surgeons, and apothecaries. By the end of the century, medical education aimed at producing a relatively uniformly trained general practitioner with dual qualifications in medicine and surgery (and, implicitly, in midwifery). All doctors were therefore firstly general practitioners; and specialist consultant training came after registration, on top of the general training. The educational by-product was 'the safe general practitioner', ready to practise independently on the day of qualification (a situation which still applies for dentistry). Naturally enough this was a major constraint on the educational philosophy (even at universities), which jettisoned most of its 'gentlemanly' humane ideals in favour of an ideal of utilitarian vocational training. As a result, the curriculum became highly prescribed — and very congested, because anything which a general practitioner 'ought' to know could be justified for inclusion. The innate conservatism of medical education is shown clearly by the fact that — despite the fact that the student no longer needs to be a competent practical doctor on graduation day, owing to the introduction of extensive, compulsory, supervised post-graduate training — examiners continue to behave as if the safe general practitioner (or perhaps the safe house officer) were the one essential goal of undergraduate training.

Far from witnessing a revolution in medical education, what we can see at work is a profound inertia, where the educational process consistently lags behind practice. By contrast, it is difficult to name any instance where educational reform has stimulated a change in practice (it remains to be seen whether the increasing percentage of women medical graduates may prove the exception).

The reasons for such conservatism become obvious when we study the power structures of the various educational establishments. The medical corporations have always acted primarily to safeguard their own (short-term) interests; which they have done very capably by means of their ancient prestige and expertise at lobbying and obstruction. This was acceptable when professional, educational, and public interests were thought to be identical; but few people would now assume that such a confluence of benefit was inevitable.

The universities have been little better at stimulating radical change. Again the inertia is formidable, although in this case it appears to be the product of an interlocking system of departmental interests which — once it has crystallized — ensures that nothing can be changed without changing everything. On top of this, there is no mechanism by which change is built into the system; on the contrary there is an assumption of the *status quo ad infinitum*.

If revolutionary change is difficult, this is also because doctors value the present system as a whole. At the bottom line it does produce enough doctors who are good enough to keep the system afloat; and they fear to throw the baby out with the bathwater. A revolution in education is bound to be expensive and time-consuming — or so it is assumed. Supposing, after all the trauma, that the revolutionary new system did not work, that the 'doctors' produced could not do the job, or were regarded as incapable or unsafe, and were despised and disregarded by conventionally-educated doctors! We will return to this question at the end of the book.

In conclusion: because there have been no revolutions in British medical education in the past we assume that there will probably be no revolutions in the future. Change, if it comes, will be gradual and piecemeal, and should be carefully assessed at each stage. That does not mean, however, that change should be random or regressive, nor that it should be directed towards inappropriate goals. The question of what goals are appropriate for the making of a doctor, and what changes in education might make these goals attainable, will engage us in subsequent chapters. In the mean time we shall look at another matter which has varied throughout history.

2.3 Duration of training

During the nineteenth century the minimum length of study, and the nature of that study, were prescribed by Act of Parliament in response to pressure from the emerging medical profession (although in practice these constraints were not rigidly enforced). Such control over entry into a given profession is actually a part of the process by which a group defines itself *as* a profession. Prolonged junior status is only partly educational in its motivation: there are also considerations of social status (who is allowed to enter the profession); academic status (what are the minimum entrance qualifications, how long must the juniors study, how difficult are their examinations); and hierarchical status within the profession (a prolonged apprenticeship is an important method by which senior doctors influence the attitudes and aptitudes of their junior colleagues).

So we may observe that, when a group is trying to enhance its status, increasing the minimum length of training is one common strategy adopted. Consider, for example, schoolteachers. Since 1945 the minimum period of study in England has doubled from two to four years, and all new teachers must be graduates (the actual effect on enhancing status has, however, not been impressive). Another example is pharmacy; despite the considerable erosion of dispensing skills resulting from factory preparation of medicines, pharmacy is now largely a graduate profession too. An interesting exception is 'the Bar', where the period of training is still relatively short. But the Bar retains its exclusivity by ensuring that the juniors are initially virtually unpaid, restricting entry to those with a 'private income'. What these examples show is that the process called 'inflation of qualifications' is not always a consequence of educational need, nor inevitable, but must be interpreted in a broader social context.

The length of medical study is partly a reflection of the requirements of practice. During the nineteenth century there was very little specialization: most doctors treated most ailments. A licence to practise was seen as a minimum enforceable level of competence, and beyond this minimum it was the responsibility of individuals to seek out whatever training they thought appropriate for whatever career they wished to pursue. This was stimulated by competition. It is important to remember that there was no guaranteed income; doctors were — if anything — overproduced, and lucrative positions were hard to obtain. There was therefore a clear financial, as well as educational, incentive to gain prestige by obtaining an impressive higher training, with references from eminent practitioners.

Our starting-point in the mid-nineteenth century is a general training of about four years designed to turn out a 'safe general practitioner': one ready, in other words, for a lifetime of practice on the day of qualification. Owing to the peculiarities of legislation it was for several decades possible to practise with *either* a medical (apothecaries' or physicians') *or* a surgical qualification — both were not essential. But the demarcation between the three 'orders' proved impossible to police in the face of both public and professional indifference, and instead the double qualification of medicine and surgery became the minimum requirement for a general practitioner (or 'surgeon apothecary'). It is worth noticing that the tendency was established early to 'improve' training by *accumulation* of qualifications, rather than by rationalizing previously established qualifications. So the psychiatrist was initially a member of the college of physicians, and a specialist surgeon had first to train as a general surgeon. That this process is not inevitable can be seen by a comparison with the USA (and several European countries), where specialist training is embarked upon immediately after the MD; and by the foundation of the new British colleges or sub-specialist qualifications, so that now a psychiatrist can acquire membership of the college of psychiatrists and the ophthalmic surgeon may be spared work as a casualty officer and varicose vein stripper.

None the less, since Victorian times the period of training has expanded by stages. Inflation of qualifications means that more and more qualifications will 'buy' the doctor less and less in career terms. Medicine has added a year to the minimum time for qualification. This now consists of the following: first, five years at university (though there are also a substantial minority of students who intercalate a B.Sc. or the equivalent, and various mature students with a range of other qualifications). Then follows a compulsory pre-registration year added in 1951 — ostensibly as an educational experience, but in actuality functioning as a source of cheap menial labour. But it is in the post-registration period that the greatest expansion of training has occurred. All medical practitioners who wish to work independently and unsupervised must now complete a minimum of three years' additional post-registration training.

In other words, the philosophy of medical education has changed from 'the safe general practitioner' ready for anything on the day of qualification, to the graduation of a kind of pluripotential 'stem'-doctor — designed as a general-purpose substrate for 'trial-by-housejob'; who is then subjected to further training towards independent practice in a variety of consultant specialties or a general practice.

This function of post-registration training has been taken on by the remnants of the old medical corporations, the Royal Colleges. These are examining bodies, whatever teaching they do being strictly optional and on a fee-for-course basis. The colleges also enjoy a great deal of autonomy in regulating their own branches of the profession: although the significance of acceptance into membership or fellowship of a college as a certificate of advanced training can be anything from the preliminary level of an MRCP after eighteen months, to the 'exit' or pre-consultant examinations of the M.R.C. Path. This autonomy and freedom from external regulation has allowed the perpetuation of numerous abuses in the nature and content of examinations (which are, however, financially profitable to the corporations). In particular, the colleges of physicians and surgeons enforce extraordinarily high percentage failure-rates, which seem arbitrary in their selectivity, but result in vast numbers of resit examinations — at a price. There also exists the somewhat anomalous situation whereby the acceptance by, and continued membership of, a college, is taken to be synonymous with competence in a specialty. Although college membership is not a legal requirement for consultant or principal GP status, in practice it is rare to succeed without such membership.

The outcome of a century and a half of inflation is that medical training has expanded from about four or five years, to a minimum of nine years for a general practitioner (usually longer), and about fifteen years for many consultant specialties. This is not just a matter of regulations, which are often surprisingly liberal, but more of the demands of the job market; doctors generally tend to overqualify themselves in order to be confident of getting the jobs they want. By such a process an initial training in general medicine culminating in the MRCP has become common as a preliminary to a wide range of 'non-physicianly' specialties such as radiology and psychiatry, some branches of pathology, and even general practice. In this sense the MRCP has almost evolved into an extension of the pre-registration year — the *preliminary* training having expanded to eight years for MB MRCP. The fact that this trend has happened 'on the nod' and is not a regulation makes it all the more difficult to criticize or evaluate — junior doctors are trying to second-guess the decisions of multiple appointment committees. This inflationary trend is exacerbated by career uncertainty (MRCP is acceptable as a high-status, general qualification, while the same amount of time spent in psychiatry or anaesthetics would not be), and by lack of clinical confidence following the educationally inadequate pre-registration year.

Increased duration of training is commonly regarded as a 'good thing' on the assumption that it is motivated and justified by educational goals. But we can see that historically this has not usually been the case; professional factors are more obvious, and financial advantage not uncommon. Consider for instance the convenience of the cheap labour of pre-registration house officers (on an hourly basis the lowest paid NHS employees), and of consultants being 'protected' from dull ward work and on-call duties by the large numbers of juniors in training.

But there are two major disadvantages of a continual expansion of the duration of training. Firstly, the professional life of the practitioner is shortened. Surgeons may be well past their peak of performance before they are appointed as consultants. This is both expensive and inefficient. Secondly, and more importantly, the public frequently finds itself being treated by junior doctors, many of whom have been doing the job for only a short time. This is exacerbated by the educationally dubious practice of short-stay (six weeks, four months, or six months) rotational training schemes which give a brief taste of every specialty. So that when patients are likely to be at their most ill — at the time of admission — they are most likely to be treated by the least experienced member of the medical hierarchy!

The requirement for prolonged training also produces inflexibility — it is very difficult to switch between specialties when it takes years to qualify in each. This has the further effect of keeping specialist-trained people hanging around gathering qualifications and experience while desperately looking for jobs. One only has to glance at the university calendar to see that no one in academic life spends more time accumulating qualifications than doctors.

But perhaps the most damning criticism of postgraduates medical education is that it is misdirected. The historical expansion of medical education from four to fourteen years has taken place entirely at the *beginning* of the doctor's career; continuing education of general practitioners and consultants remains in its infancy. It is easy to see how this has happened. With the medical corporations in the hands of the senior practitioners, postgraduate education has been merely a matter of erecting more and higher hurdles for junior doctors to jump, before being allowed to join 'the bosses', while the bosses have omitted to set up hurdles for themselves . . . Yet it is the educational deficiencies of older practitioners which can sometimes be the problem, rather than those of their over-qualified and immensely experienced senior registrars and GP trainees! It is a question of directing educational effort to where it is needed for educational reasons, and for knowing when the point of diminishing returns has been reached, and passed.

For these reasons we believe that continuing medical education is in need of reform, in contrast with the training of junior doctors, which is, by and large, pretty effective already, and more often than not bloated beyond the point of need. We shall have more to say on this matter in the section devoted to continuing medical education.

2.4   The General Medical Council

The General Medical Council was established as a result of the Medical Act of 1858, and in some ways its role today remains heavily influenced by the specific and historical circumstances surrounding its inception.

Until recently, the 1858 Act was regarded as a landmark in medical progress. It was seen as unifying the medical profession for the first time, and as regulating both education and ethical behaviour in the public interest. But a more critical examination has revealed that the Act is more plausibly interpreted as a prime example of professional self-interest in action, with the medical corporations (especially the colleges of physicians and surgeons) hijacking the movement towards reform in order to bolster up their entrenched privileges. The medical profession was not unified by the Act, and medical education was left virtually unchanged.

The 1858 Act followed at least fifteen attempts to frame legislation in medical Bills during the preceding years. The medical reformers wanted four major changes; a definition of medical qualification, a register of qualified doctors, the rationalization of medical education and examinations, and a regulatory medical council to run the show. These goals were combined in the desire for a 'single portal of entry' to medicine; a single qualification regulated by state examinations.

Need for reform in the public interest was formulated against a background of approximately eighteen degree-, diploma-, and licentiate-awarding institutions, with variable and incompatible standards of entry and tests of proficiency. Some institutions awarded their certificates as a blatantly commercial activity, with hardly any pretence of rigour — rather like the bogus correspondence colleges of today. There was no consensus as to which qualifications were recognized where, and highly competent practitioners often operated under threat of prosecution by institutions attempting to enforce ancient monopolies (for example, even superbly trained Scottish graduates were, for a while, not allowed to practise in London).

The 1858 Act followed hard on the heels of the successful thwarting of plans to establish a college of general practitioners, in which the colleges of physicians and surgeons were once again the villains. The final form of the Act demonstrated the corporations' dislike of any change which threatened their health and wealth, and demonstrated too their power to prevent change. The eventual constitution of the GMC with a heavy majority of corporation and university members ensured that the spectre of GP influence was held in check for many years to come. Other major aims of the reformers were a determination to outlaw 'quackery' (medical practice by the unqualified), and also to ban the practice of what might now be called 'alternative' medical systems such as homoeopathy. But, with the later exception of a ban on unqualified practitioners treating venereal disease (!), such prohibition has never been achieved in the UK. Quackery is legal, although quacks are not allowed to claim that they are medically qualified when they are not.

But in terms of medical education the Medical Act was a resounding failure. The Act defined 'medical qualification' so widely that it was perfectly legal to practise surgery after training in medicine alone (or *vice versa*); there was no significant rationalization of the number of institutions or statutory harmonization of standards; and large numbers of established but unqualified practitioners were admitted to the register.

Many of these abuses and irregularities were gradually reformed during the century, although more by professional evolution and 'market forces' than by statutory requirement. The statutory requirement for qualifications in both medicine and surgery, together with midwifery, had to wait nearly thirty years, until the Amendment Act of 1886. Only once did the

GMC withdraw its recognition of a qualification from an institution — in the case of the Apothecaries Hall of Dublin in 1895. But the 'single portal of entry' to the medical profession has never been established. Students who have failed their university examinations and are (presumably) regarded by their *alma mater* as unfit to practise medicine, are still able to attempt the conjoint, triple, or Apothecaries' licentiate examinations which are offered by the corporations (exams almost universally regarded as being set at a considerably lower standard than the medical degree). The fact that this bizarre 'loophole' is still left open is something of an anachronism, although the competitive nature of junior medical appointments prevents the situation's being widely abused (students are understandably reluctant to signal to their colleagues that they have failed to obtain university qualifications).

So, what has been the role of the GMC with regard to medical education? This is a difficult question to answer, not least because no historian has tackled the subject. While the GMC had undoubtedly exerted a powerful, although unquantifiable, 'deterrent' effect on unethical conduct, its effect on education has been much less certain. As was stated above, it has only once used actual compulsion in order to prevent a gross insufficiency in qualifying exams. Anecdotal evidence suggests that its influence 'behind the scenes' may indeed have been considerable; and of course the GMC was able to influence the establishment of new medical schools (most recently Southampton, Nottingham, and Leicester) in a more overt fashion.

But the influence of the GMC is limited by its legal powers. Its only statutory weapon is the Draconian measure of refusing to recognize a licence, diploma, or degree, which is far too extreme a measure for the purpose of encouraging the gradual and considered reform of medical education. On the other hand, it has the right to visit medical schools and also to inspect their examinations, which gives the GMC a unique and privileged insight into medical education nationally. The GMC visit is in itself a considerable deterrent, as the preparations will involve an institution in considerable extra work, and the threat of a further inspection if matters are unsatisfactory has a similar impact. Moreover the GMC publishes Recommendations on Basic Medical Education (for example 1967 and 1978, with another currently in preparation) which are (in our opinion) full of good ideas and insightful analysis. However, it has no way to ensure that these recommendations are even read, let alone implemented!

Furthermore, the GMC has a role in regulating postgraduate education. This includes the pre-registration year (for which their recommendations have been almost completely ignored); the 'recognition' of additional qualifications for registration, such as higher degrees and corporation memberships (this is merely a rubber-stamping exercise); and the 'co-ordination of all stages of medical education' to quote the constitution, which includes specialist and continuing medical education. In other words the remit covers the whole of medical education from admission to medical school right through to retirement from practice.

It is clear that the GMC has a vast potential for good in medical education. But on the other hand, it lacks teeth; the weapon of refusing to recognize qualifications is far too crude for the purpose of stimulating reform. The GMC has, for example, failed to prevent the decline of the pre-registration housejob to its current dire state. What is more, the old corporations have maintained their stranglehold on specialist examinations (and therefore education) with an *increase* in the fragmentation of training. As we write the colleges of London, Edinburgh, and Glasgow are once again refusing to recognize each other's Part One surgical examinations — a return to the bad old days with a vengeance. The upshot is that surgeons must pay to repeat the same examination in more than one college. Profitable, no doubt, but educationally unjustifiable.

It is perhaps unfair to complain that the GMC has not done more. After all, it operates pretty much on a shoestring, and mostly in the spare time of busy and active clinicians. Nevertheless, it is all we have to prevent abuses and maintain educational standards. And on the evidence of the GMC Recommendations it is clear that both the knowledge and the will are already present, and it is simply a matter of getting the medical schools, hospitals, and corporations to take notice. It is possible, although unlikely, that the statutory powers of the GMC could be extended by Act of Parliament, so that people would be literally forced to take notice. But there are other options.

There is little doubt that the GMC is accorded a high level of respect by the profession and the public. What the GMC says has influence. Currently its pronouncements are framed, as they have always been, in careful mandarin prose, couched in general terms, concerned with only the broadest of recommendations, and designed — as gently as possible — to build a moderate consensus. However, if we compare the Recommendations with the actuality, we must conclude that this is patently not enough to bring about reform. What then can be done?

One suggestion is that the GMC should name names! This would — we suspect — act as a serious deterrent to transgressors. By a combination of inspections (repeated if necessary) and public dissemination of reports, the GMC should be quite explicit just when and how an institution is failing to educate its students in an appropriate manner. The worst offenders should be made an example of. No medical school would wish to be singled out for the criticism of the GMC. A health authority which exploited its house officers would not enjoy having the fact broadcast to the media with the full authority of the Council. The threat and actuality of publishing the 'names and addresses' of the perpetrators of bad educational practice would undoubtedly act as a powerful incentive to give serious consideration to GMC recommendations. At the very least it would ensure that any counter-arguments were water-tight.

Such a proposal may seem in direct contrast to the principle of professional etiquette that no doctor should publicly criticize another. But this injunction does not apply to institutions. And if the GMC does not have the right of criticism, then who does? Who else will defend the overall interests of medical education against the power of vested interest? We would encourage the GMC to explore ways to ensure that its Recommendations, into which so much expertise and effort have been poured, will not simply be ignored by the universities and the corporations.

2.5 Conclusions

1. Medical education is profoundly influenced by its history.

2. It has evolved in a piecemeal fashion, without revolutions, and with a continued tendency to hold on to its past even when this is not appropriate.

3. Left to their own devices, there is a tendency for the universities and medical corporations to act in their own best interests, rather than those of good education.

4. The GMC has an essential role in encouraging and, when necessary, enforcing high standards of practice across the whole range of medical education. Such a role requires expansion of the Council's activities.

Bibliography

General Medical Council (1985). *Centenary of the General Medical Council 1858–1958*. GMC, London.

Louden, I. (1986). *Medical care and the general practitioner 1750–1850*. Oxford University Press.

Newman, C. (1957). *The evolution of medical education in the nineteenth century*. Oxford University Press.

Poynter, F. N. L. (1966). *The evolution of medical education in Britain*. Pitman, London.

3 Aims and aptitudes: what is the good doctor good at?

3.1 Some cases

Consider the following imaginary cases, or vignettes:

3.1.1

Dr D is a GP who was very successful at medical school. He has just seen a patient who complained of sleeping problems. On asking whether she had any worries he was eventually told that she was not happy in her marriage and had fallen in love with another teacher in the school at which she taught. She wanted to explain her problems in more detail, but Dr D felt unable to help and just a little embarrassed. He prescribed sleeping pills, but was worried as to whether he had done the right thing. After some hesitation about confidentiality he asked the advice of his older partner. The partner made a tasteless remark and said 'We're doctors, not marriage counsellors.' Dr D felt a little better, but was still uneasy.

3.1.2

Mr F is a surgeon who has just had a row with a patient's relatives. He has successfully carried out an operation. But the operation involved a number of possible side-effects. He explained these to the patient. The relatives are now alleging that the patient did not understand what was being said.

3.1.3

Dr I is an SHO who did well at Medical School and spent a year as a JHO in top hospitals. The registrar and consultant in his present post have left him with a reasonable amount of responsibility. He makes a decision on one patient, and to his surprise the ward sister tells him that she thinks his decision is the wrong one. Dr I is not accustomed to having his views questioned by nurses, and when he consults the registrar he is told that the sister is very experienced and should be listened to, and that the issues should be raised at the team meeting. Dr I secretly disapproves, because he is firmly of the opinion that nurses totally lack his scientific training.

3.1.4

Dr S is irritated to read in his local newspaper that a health education officer has been appointed to try to improve the health of his neighbourhood, where the rate of smoking-related disease is high. He regards the appointment as a waste of money: 'Health education is my responsibility. All my patients have been warned by me against smoking.'

3.2 Roles, skills, and aims

The problems which we tried to highlight in the foregoing vignettes arise out of confusion in the idea of what a doctor ought to be doing at the present time. We must therefore consider the concept of a doctor. Such a concept is not an unchanging idea. Whereas there is a historical and cultural continuity in the concept of a doctor, so that we can still recognize the preoccupations of Hippocrates or Galen as those of a doctor in our sense, there is no doubt that there are also historical developments and cultural differences. We shall be concerned with the doctor in Western culture at the end of the twentieth century. How can the job of a doctor be described?

Occupations can be described or classified from three different points of view, or in terms of three different sets of concepts: as role-jobs, skill-jobs, and aim-jobs. For example, the jobs of income tax inspector or mayor are role-jobs, 'role' here being defined in terms of a set of rights and duties. In contrast, the job of musician is defined in terms of a skill, or a set of skills — to be a musician one must logically have certain skills. This is not to say that certain skills are not in fact required for the job of a mayor or an income tax inspector to be carried out successfully; but it is to say that an adequate definition of those jobs need contain no reference to these skills. On the other hand, a reference to the relevant skills is logically required for an adequate definition of the jobs of a musician or a plumber; we can claim that the statement 'Hamish is a musician/plumber' is essentially connected with the statement 'Hamish is skilled at music/plumbing.' In general, the distinction between role-jobs and skill-jobs can be stated as follows: the connection between a skill-job and the possession of an ability is a logical one, whereas the connection between a role-job and the possession of an ability is a pragmatic one — a person may in practice need certain skills in order to acquire a role-job or to perform it well, but possessing the skills is not part of the definition of the job.

Let us now turn to aim-jobs. It would seem to be the case that a number of occupations are defined in terms of some end or aim. For example, the job of 'farmer' can be said to be an aim-job, in that to be a farmer is to aim at cultivation, milk or beef production, or whatever. Similarly, the job of 'forester' is defined in terms of an aim; and so also is the job of 'game-keeper'. It is not necessary that the aim should always be attained, and obviously skill in the choosing and implementing of means will have a bearing here; but before people can be described as farmers, foresters, gamekeepers, and so on they must at least see themselves as aiming at certain ends. We would call people bad farmers if they chose the wrong means to those ends, or were unskilful at implementing the means; but if they are not pursuing those ends at all then they are not farmers. The same would hold for all who profess occupations which are aim-jobs. In general, then, to say that A, B, or C is an aim-job, is to say that there exists some purpose, aim, or end which is logically connected with job A, B, or C. It is to say that unless people have the aims in question, they cannot be counted as members of the class of those who have jobs A, B or C.

We have tended to speak so far as if there were three types of job, and this is so in the sense that some jobs are to be defined in terms of one or other of the three categories of role, aim, or skill. And it is also so irrespective of the fact that many jobs, while they may be *defined* in one of the three ways, clearly involve the other categories also. In the case of some jobs, however, it is not so obvious that they are to be defined in one category rather than another, and at any rate they certainly involve all three. The job of teacher is one example of this. For 'teacher' cannot be defined exclusively by reference to any one of the three categories, but requires to be placed in all three. Similarly, and importantly for our purposes, the job of 'doctor' cannot be placed in any single one of these categories, but requires to be defined in terms of all three. Note that this is not just making the point that being a doctor happens to be describable in terms of all three characteristics, while belonging mainly to one of the three categories — as being a mayor might involve having aims and skills, but be essentially a role-job. The point is that the job of being a doctor, like that of being a teacher, must be seen in terms of all three categories, or serious distortion or bias in medical education will result. To bring this out let us consider medicine first in terms of its aims. What is the aim of the doctor?

3.3 'Doctor' as an aim-job

It might be objected immediately that there is no one aim of the doctor; different doctors have different aims and one and the same doctor may have many aims. We can make a start in dealing with this complexity by distinguishing, as is done in many medical and other contexts, between aims and objectives. Let us say that an aim of the doctor is to try to promote health. It will follow that the doctor will have many specific objectives which are generated by the broader aim. This distinction helps, but still leaves complexities in need of conceptual tidying. We therefore need to draw a few distinctions in the concept of aim as it applies to a doctor.

In the first place, a person who happens to be a doctor will have various aims which are not necessarily connected with his occupation, although they are furthered by it. Let us call these his 'personal aims'. For example, he might aim at earning his living, at having job security, or at expressing his idealism. These are legitimately regarded as among his aims as a doctor, in that he fulfils them by means of his occupation, but they are not connected with his occupation as such, since they might just as easily be satisfied by other occupations. Hence they can be identified as 'personal aims'. Note that it does not follow from the fact that they are not connected with medicine as such that they are unimportant, or that they should be disregarded in medical education. Indeed, it may be that job satisfaction or dissatisfaction are in fact largely connected with the opportunities of the doctor to fulfil his personal aims through the practice of medicine.

Secondly, and most importantly, there is what we shall call the 'intrinsic aim' of the doctor, the aim which must logically be entertained by the doctor *qua* doctor. We shall state here quite briefly what must later be elaborated: that the intrinsic aim of the doctor is the promotion of health in its broadest sense. We shall later specify the relevant senses of 'health' and of 'promotion'. To say this is not, of course, to say that only doctors have this aim — other occupations, such as nurses and other branches of the 'caring' professions, also entertain this intrinsic aim. But it is to make health, or the relief of suffering, or healing, the intrinsic aim of the doctor.

It may be objected, however, that doctors sometimes have other aims, or other objectives, which cannot easily be put under this heading, such as certifying that someone is suitable for a certain job, or reporting that a given refuse dump constitutes a health hazard. To reply to this type of objection we require a third category of aim.

The third category of aim we shall call the 'extrinsic aim' of the doctor. To ask about the extrinsic aim of the doctor is to ask not so much about what he might achieve *in* the practice of medicine but *as a result of it*, meaning by that the indirect or non-medical consequence of it. For example, as a result of his medical practice a doctor might hope to promote health in the community, say by making public statements on the dangers of addictive drugs, or on the need to have adequate facilities for recreation, or on access to public places for the disabled. These are legitimate and desirable aims, which at least some doctors might pursue as a result of their medical education; but they are not the concerns of the doctor *qua* doctor, or so we are asserting.

We are insisting on this to prevent the concept of the doctor's becoming so wide that no education, however intensive or long-lasting, could ever qualify a person to become one. There are many competing and conflicting demands on the time of doctors; but we must distinguish what is intrinsic to their activities from what they can sometimes do as a result of their skills and role in society.

It should be noted, to avoid confusion, that what we have been contrasting as the intrinsic and extrinsic aims of the doctor can also be expressed in terms of the intrinsic and extrinsic aims of medicine. Using the term 'medicine' we might make the desired contrast by opposing aims *in* medicine (what medicine essentially consists of) with aims *for* medicine (the use which might be made of medicine by, for example, insurance companies or other bodies). We shall adopt either terminology as it may be convenient in various contexts.

3.4 Health as an aim

To maintain, as we have done, that the intrinsic aim of medicine is health is uncontroversial, to the extent that it is too vague to quarrel with. What do we mean by health? There has been a large amount of writing on the concept of health in the last ten years, and out of that literature there has emerged a complex view of health in which we can distinguish various elements. The first of these is often called 'negative health', or the absence of ill-health. 'Ill-health' itself is a complex notion, comprising disease, illness, handicap, injury, and other related ideas. These overlapping concepts can be linked if they are seen on the model of abnormal, unwanted, or incapacitating states of a biological system. Sometimes negative health is called the 'bio-medical model' of health.

Secondly, the idea of 'positive health' has more recently appeared in published reports. The origins of this idea are in the definition of health to be found in the preamble to the Constitution of the World Health Organization (WHO): 'Health is a state of complete physical, mental and social well-being, and not merely the absence of disease or infirmity.' (WHO 1946).

It follows from this definition that 'well-being' is an important ingredient in positive health. 'Well-being' is a complex concept, and it is important in this context to distinguish well-being as a subjective mood or state from the well-being which is rooted in life-style. In the first sense, a mood of well-being can be induced by drugs or alcohol. This may sometimes be a good thing, and sometimes doctors might prescribe drugs which induce it on a temporary basis to enable someone to recover from a depression. In the second sense, well-being comes from a life-style based on friends, interests, a reasonable diet, and some exercise. The lack of adequate discussion of this, the most important sense of well-being, is a serious omission in many medical courses. There is a third side to well-being, which we shall discuss shortly, but shall mention here for the sake of completeness. This side is often expressed through the concept of 'welfare'. There is no one meaning of well-being in this third sense, but it is convenient to think of a person's welfare as being the aspects of his/her well-being which are affected by such matters as housing, employment, environment, etc.

A third idea in the concept of health is that of 'fitness'. Fitness in its most obvious sense refers to the state of someone's heart and lungs. To be fit in this sense is to have a place on a scale ranging from being able to climb stairs or run for a bus without getting out of breath to being able to run a marathon or climb Mount Everest. Fitness can also be used in a related but broader sense, which we might call the 'sociological' as opposed to the 'heart and lungs' sense. In the sociological sense of fitness a person is fit *for* some occupation or job. This means that people have the necessary health to enable them to perform their job or task adequately without, for example, too many days off work.

It is tempting to think of fitness as standing alongside well-being as a component in positive health. But this is a mistake; fitness can be seen as part of either the negative or the positive dimensions of health. We are healthy in the negative sense if we are not ill or diseased; analogously we can be fit in the negative sense if we can manage to perform the tasks of daily life — stair-climbing, walking to and fro, luggage-lifting, and so on — without undue physical stress. The analogue to positive well-being is the fitness which enables a person to swim, ride a bicycle, climb a hill, and so on. Fitness, then, is best seen as a component of both negative and positive health rather than as a separate dimension to health.

The WHO definition refers to the 'mental and social' as well as to the physical. Nevertheless, the mental and social components of health are the poor relations of the health services and do not receive adequate attention in published reports, or adequate funding from governments or research institutions. Moreover, to begin with mental health, it is certainly true that mental health is most often taken to be the absence of mental ill-health. A case can be made for the existence of a positive dimension to mental health. The danger of this is that it might encourage conformity or fitting in with prevailing social norms and attitudes; but there are ways of looking at positive mental health which avoid this charge.

The idea of 'social well-being' is in fact just as obscure as that of mental well-being, although at first sight it does not seem to be a difficult notion. What does it mean? In one sense 'social well-being' refers to the skills and other abilities which enable us to form friendships and relate to other people in conversation and through the many different sorts of contacts which are part of ordinary social life. Sometimes these are called 'lifeskills', and the possession of them helps to create a sense of 'self-esteem', which is currently a fashionable concept in the literature of health education. Clearly, like fitness, social well-being in this sense can be graded on a scale from negative to positive. It is a property of individuals and refers to their ability to cope in a social context — hence 'social well-being' is an appropriate term.

But does it make sense to speak of 'social well-being' in a stricter sense — one which makes the well-being a characteristic of society itself, as distinct from the individuals who are in society? One way of making sense of this idea is to think of society not in terms of the individuals who make it up, but in terms of the institutions, practices, customs, political arrangements, social class relationships, and so on, which give structure to the society. From this point of view people are related to each other by the structures of their society, and indeed part of their identity is created by these social structures. We could then evaluate a society in terms of the way in which its social structures tend to produce well-being in the people who belong to that society. Just as we sometimes praise the 'atmosphere' in a school or hospital as one of well-being, so the social structures of an entire society might be said to make for or detract from well-being.

Some theorists with firm attachments to empiricism might prefer to understand what we have said as referring to health determinants rather than health itself. For example, they might agree that a society with marked social class gradients and corresponding gradients in the distribution of ill-health is one with a tendency to create ill-health in individuals. Thus, in terms of this approach, if we speak of an 'unhealthy society' we are simply speaking metaphorically about the determinants, such as poor housing, diet, and so on, that have helped to produce poor health states in individuals. Other thinkers might maintain that it is not a metaphor to characterize social relationships and structures as being themselves unhealthy. It is perhaps self-indulgent to pursue this theoretical question here.

It is not self-indulgent, however, to examine the relationship between health negatively and health positively conceived. Can we link the absence of ill-health and the presence of well-being in a single concept of health in the manner of the WHO definition? This is not a rarefied question, because it affects the legitimate scope of medicine. If well-being is a component in the concept of health then clearly medicine has a much wider remit than it would otherwise have.

One important factor influencing this question is that ill-health and well-being cannot be related to each other as opposite poles on a linear scale. This approach has been tried by some theorists, but it is not satisfactory, for it is logically possible (and not in fact uncommon) for someone to have poor physical health but a high state of well-being — as in the case of a terminal patient in a hospice who is supported by a caring staff and loving friends — or a good state of physical health but poor well-being — as in the case of someone who has no diseases or illnesses but lacks friends, a job, interests.

The fact that health (the absence of ill-health) and well-being cannot be related on a linear scale must raise the question of whether they are in fact two components of a single concept. It may be preferable and less confusing conceptually to think of them as two overlapping concepts rather than as a single concept with two dimensions. Thus the feeling of well-being that a person has after an invigorating swim can fairly be described as a 'glow of health', but the well-being or satisfaction that a person has after writing a chapter in a book, listening to a piece of music, or just playing a diverting game is less obviously related to the concept of health, and more obviously related to concepts such as 'enjoyment', 'happiness', etc. Again, the well-being that is created by moving someone to better housing is more obviously related to the concept of 'welfare' than to that of health. The conclusion is that while the concepts of health and well-being overlap they are distinct and cannot be combined into one concept.

It does not of course follow from the fact that well-being is a different concept from health that medicine has no bearing on it. To take analogous cases, a doctor might reasonably be concerned with the processes of aging, or with contraception.

But neither getting older as such nor pregnancy constitutes ill-health. In other words, the legitimate activities of a doctor may be wider than coping with ill-health.

It is helpful here to use the distinction we drew earlier between the intrinsic and the extrinsic aim of the doctor. The intrinsic aim of the doctor is the improvement of health in the negative sense — the removal of ill-health. But a doctor may also have the extrinsic aim of furthering positive health in the sense of the well-being and welfare of his/her patients. As we said, a doctor is well-placed to join social workers, health educationists, and others to further positive health. To see this as a doctor's extrinsic aim is not to undervalue positive health but to assign priorities; a doctor's education cannot fit him/her for every task, and we suggest that the promotion of negative health (the bio-medical model) is the intrinsic aim, and the promotion of positive health is the extrinsic aim.

The distinction, between the intrinsic and the extrinsic aim of the doctor, or between the aims of the doctor and those of the health education officer, or between negative and positive health, is sufficiently important to be worth taking further. We can develop the distinction by comparing medicine with health education. What is the function of health education?

At a very general level we can answer the question by a broad statement of aim: *Health education is an activity aimed at restoring, maintaining, or enhancing the health of individuals and communities.* This definition is not adequate, however, for it provides at best a necessary and not a sufficient definition of health education. The definition as stated could apply to the work of the doctor. Doctors of course see themselves as health educators; but in their characteristic work in pursuing their intrinsic aim, they are concerned not with education but with treatment. How then can we distinguish the work of the health educator from that of the doctor?

There are various important differences in assumption and approach. To state these is not necessarily to state a preference for one or the other. The activities are complementary and over-lap and, as has already been said, the doctor can at times act as a health educator. Nevertheless, there are differences. But before listing these we must first dispel one confusion.

It is sometimes suggested that medicine deals with scientific fact whereas health education deals with advice and exhortation; one deals with the 'is' and the other with the 'ought'. This is not true. Medicine is based on the sciences, but it also deals with advice and with prescriptions. Health education likewise advises and counsels; but it is also based on the biological and social sciences. What then are the genuine differences?

First, medicine characteristically bypasses our rational minds and treats us as causal mechanisms. This is mainly so even if the doctor also listens to the patient's 'stories'. In other words, characteristic medical treatments are biochemical or surgical, whereas health education attempts to get us to understand our bodies and their environment. Secondly, medicine typically (but again by no means exclusively) stresses the curative or palliative, whereas health education stresses the preventive. Going along with the second distinction we might say, thirdly, that medicine stresses the doctor–patient or one-to-one relationship, whereas health education tends to have a broader societal perspective. Fourthly, and perhaps most fundamentally, medicine tends to be reductivist in its assumptions — this follows from the scientific study of disease processes on which it is based — whereas health education tends to be holistic in its assumptions.

Does it follow from the distinctions, if they contain at least some truth, that health education is in some way ethically superior to medicine? This by no means follows. If I break a leg I do not want advice but treatment! In other words, there is a place for both approaches. Moreover, as we have said, some doctors may also pursue health education, and this is a legitimate aim: but it is an extrinsic aim.

It is worth noting here, what we shall shortly develop at some length, that although the intrinsic aim of the doctor is health negatively and narrowly conceived, that aim can be pursued within the broader perspective of 'whole-person understanding'. The theme of 'whole-person understanding' needs and will receive considerable analysis; but we mention it here to prevent misunderstanding. Even although the intrinsic aim of the doctor is to be seen in terms of the 'bio-medical' model of health, that aim can be successfully pursued only through whole-person care.

3.5 'Doctor' as a role-job

Medicine, in common with other professions, is a role-job, and an account of this role must be included in any adequate description of what it is to be a doctor, and hence of how doctors should be educated. Professions must be seen as role-jobs because they provide a service for other persons. Now many occupations, such as those involved in transport or public health, provide a service; but in the professions the service is provided specially via a *relationship* between the professional and his clients. What is here meant by a 'relationship'?

We can use the word 'relationship' in two ways; to stand for the bond which links two or more people, or to stand for the attitudes which bonded people have to each other. As examples of the first kind of relationship we might mention kinship, marriage, business association, or the teacher–pupil relationship. As examples of the second kind we might mention fear, pride, respect, envy, contempt, etc. Thus someone seeing an adult with a child might ask 'What is the relationship between those two?', and receive an answer in terms of the first kind of relationship: 'teacher and pupil', 'father and son', etc. Or the question might be 'What sort of relationship do Jones and his son have?', and receive an answer in terms of the second kind of relationship: 'Jones loves his son, but his son can't stand him.'

The two kinds of relationship are connected in various complex ways. For example, if the situation is a business transaction then the attitude of the parties would not characteristically be one, say, of affection or friendship. There is of course no logical impediment to such an attitude's developing out of the business transaction, and indeed it is material for romantic comedy when the attitude in the relationship is inappropriate for the bond. What, then, are the special characteristics of the doctor–patient relationship?

Let us begin by anatomizing the attitude aspect of the relationship. To understand an attitude we must consider its object. The object of the professional attitude is the patient or client conceived in terms of vulnerability; typically there is inequality of power. This is obviously the case in a doctor–patient or teacher–pupil relationship. It can be argued that because of the dominant position which doctors occupy in the relationship with their patients, and because as doctors they must supply a service, and often assess its success as well, they must be governed more than many other people by principles of ethics; in particular in this context they must be governed by a desire to be of assistance to their patients — an attitude that is often called 'beneficence'.

The inequality of the professional relationship not only requires a special attitude, it also requires a special 'bond', which usually takes the form of an institutional role-relationship. The need for a formal bond in addition to an appropriate attitude is evident if we consider the significant interventions which doctors can make in the lives of their patients. We can approach this point in another way. We have already characterized the doctor as someone who aims at health. It follows that the doctor's activities intimately bear on human good and harm, and therefore the State will take an interest in them. For example, the State will lay down broad conditions for the qualifications of doctors, or specify when a patient has a legal right to medical care, to hospitalization, and so on. There may even be cases, perhaps of certain infectious disorders or psychiatric disorders, where the doctor has a duty to commit the patient to care against his wishes. In the latter case, the authority by which a person may be compulsorily detained in a hospital in Britain is legally derived from an Act of Parliament.

The professional bond is constituted, secondly, by rather vaguer sets of rules, or even of expectations, which doctors and patients have of each other. Doctors often refer to this as the 'ethics' of their professions. There are many different facets to this. For example, a patient has the assurance that a doctor will not take advantage of him with respect to any information about his private life which emerges; and there will be no gossip about medical conditions, social predicaments, and so on. The medical profession is very strict about enforcing its own discipline on these matters.

It is important that the doctor–patient relationship should be constituted, at least partly, by these legal and quasi-legal institutional bonds, for at least the following reasons. Firstly, because doctors and all health and welfare workers, by the nature of their jobs, intervene in existentially crucial ways in the lives of others. This is a serious matter, and its consequences for a patient can be enormous. It is therefore in the interests of patients that there should be some sort of professional entitlement to intervene. In other words, if he is not simply to be a busybody, a doctor must have the *right to intervene*, and if he has the right to intervene he must have duties and responsibilities; the concept of an institution encapsulates these ideals of rights, duties, and responsibilities.

A second reason is that doctors must ask about many intimate details of people's lives, for example, about their marriages; and they also may conduct examinations of people's bodies. Questioning of this sort, and even more so physical examination, can create situations in which people can be exploited, or which could be embarrassing even to doctors themselves. The fact that it is an institutional bond which brings doctors together with their patients provides *emotional insulation* for both parties in such situations. Moreover, there must be some assurance that no untoward use will be made of the information, that it will not be passed on to neighbours, etc. But the idea of an institution entails that of rules; and the rules can, thirdly, impose *confidentiality* on the doctor, and thus provide security for the patient.

Fourthly, doctors are given a measure of *security* by virtue of the fact that they work inside an institutional framework. There are various aspects to this. For instance, it is good for all professions to have ways and means whereby new skills and knowledge can be shared, and in general whereby members of a profession can support and encourage each other. Again, doctors require legal or similar professional protection from exploitation, unfair criticism, or legal action against them by their patients. Reciprocally, there must be some institutional mechanism whereby the professions can criticize themselves and look for ways of improving their services to the public. These, then, are some of the reasons for which a complex legal and institutional structure has grown up governing directly and indirectly the relationships between health and welfare workers and their patients.

There are various desirable and undesirable aspects to this; but the relevant point for present purposes is that when the doctor, nurse, or other health worker appears to be acting as an individual he/she is also acting as a *representative* of his/her profession, and to a lesser extent also his/her State. In other words, the individual action of a doctor or other health worker expresses also the collective values of his/her profession; individual responsibility becomes collective responsibility, since it is through the individuals that their professions are represented. We might say that individual health workers represent their professions in two senses. First, they are its ascriptive representatives, in that the profession authorizes their actions, having sanctioned their training. Second, they represent the values of the profession in so far as they act in terms of its ethics, and its ethics are all-pervasive in the actions and attitudes of the individual health worker.

In sum then, the doctor-patient relationship requires the doctor to have a certain attitude — beneficence towards the vulnerability of patients; but it also requires the institutional bonds which we have described by means of the concept of a role.

We have so far used the concept of a role as a way of linking a profession as an institution with the interests of *specific* patients; but it also enables us to refer to a broader social function, which involves the duty to speak out with authority on matters of social justice and social utility. Previously we have been concerned with the duty of the doctor to help and to be fair and honest to individuals, but now we are concerned with these duties in a wider social context. A good example of this from another profession is that provided by judges when in giving judgement they also comment on the need for changes in or additions to the law, or they comment on the practices of bureaucrats or the social services. Again, doctors have a duty to speak out on broad issues of health, as for example, they might speak out against cigarette advertising. Doctors are here pursuing what we have called the 'extrinsic' aim of medicine. In this kind of way the professions can be seen to have the important social function of regulators in the interest of general utility and justice. This is another aspect of a doctor's role. The existence of this function is recognized by the practice of including doctors on some government inquiries or arbitration panels. To some extent they are invited for their expertise; but it is also because they are recognized as having this wider function as public commentators. In exercising this wider function they are pursuing what we called the 'extrinsic' aim of medicine.

Professions are legitimized by the law. Yet legal legitimacy does not fully explain the social status of a professional role; for this we must also employ the idea of 'moral legitimacy'. If a profession is to have credibility in the eyes of the general public it must be widely recognized as being independent, disciplined by its professional association, actively expanding its knowledge-base, and concerned with the education of its members. If it is widely recognized as satisfying such conditions then it will possess moral as well as legal legitimacy, and its pronouncements will be listened to with respect; it will have legitimized the authority of its role.

3.6 'Doctor' as a skill-job

The most obvious feature of medicine is its knowledge-base and its resultant skills. Indeed, the professions generally have traditionally been thought to be the custodians of special accumulations of esoteric knowledge. This does not mean that a profession is based exclusively on one discipline — on the contrary, professions tend to be eclectic, and to draw from various disciplines. This condition, a base of knowledge and resultant skills, is clearly no more than a necessary condition for being a profession, for there are many occupations which have a solid knowledge-base but which are not professions. For example, a systems analyst, or a film director, and many others, have considerable knowledge and skills — more than many professionals are likely to have; but their occupations are not professions. On the other hand the condition does rule out some occupations which are claiming professional status. For example, the knowledge and skills involved in, say, estate agency or advertising do not seem sufficient to qualify these occupations for entry into the professions through that route, although they may have other attributes in common with some of the professions.

Let us now look in more detail at the knowledge and skills involved in medicine.

Each one within the broad range of the health care professions will have its own particular knowledge-base, although there will be a large amount of overlap. For example, whereas a medical student requires a fairly comprehensive and general knowledge of anatomy and physiology, a speech therapist or a dentist needs a far more detailed knowledge of the anatomy and physiology of the mouth and related areas. It would also be prudent for all health care workers to acquire some knowledge of the law to the extent that it bears on their professional work.

In clinical terms examples of the factual knowledge of doctors would include such pieces of information as:

The blood is pumped by the heart to the arteries, the arterioles, and the capillaries and returns in the venous system to be oxygenated in the lungs.

Cimetidine is an H_2 receptor antagonist and reduces gastric acid secretion.

These are simple clinical facts. Yet in a historical sense it is important to note that such information was not always available, and that in the future new answers and facts will inevitably come to light which may change our whole concept of a particular disease or illness.

It is important to recognize that changing the factual knowledge may change the kinds of decision that have to be made. Take the introduction of cimetidine for example. Prior to this the management of chronic duodenal ulceration was by simple symptomatic measures such as bed rest or antacids, or by a surgical procedure. The decision as to when to operate was a difficult one. The introduction of cimetidine as an effective non-operative technique for controlling the disease changed the balance of decisions, and introduced a wider choice for the patient and the doctor.

Since doctors are practical people, their primary aim is doing rather than knowing. But practical skills or *knowledge how* require a factual substrate or knowledge-base which is essential for the development of practical skills. Arising from a broad factual knowledge-base there will be a huge range of professional skills, from the simple knowing how to take blood to the more complex knowing how to bypass coronary arteries.

In addition to the practical skills originating in their factual knowledge-bases all health care professions require skills in communicating effectively with their patients or clients. Most training programmes now include some explicit study of and practice in communications skills, which traditionally have been learned by apprenticeship.

Like factual knowledge, practical skills are constantly changing and improving. One has only to look at recent developments in health care, transplantation, *in vitro* fertilization, coronary artery bypass procedures, bone marrow transplantation, vaccination against hepatitis, to see how these practical skills may change our views on life expectancy and challenge our traditional values. New procedures and skills will continually evolve, and the doctor, nurse, or other health care professional must constantly be updating skills in diagnosis, prevention, screening, and treatment. We shall discuss this important matter of updating skills in Chapter 10.

3.7 Teams

Traditionally doctors have thought of themselves as working on their own, with perhaps support from some others, especially nurses. This is increasingly an unrealistic idea. Health-care is now delivered by teams, and this is true in general practice as well as in hospitals. The concept of a team is one which combines the concepts in terms of which we have been characterizing the profession of a doctor. Thus teams in health care have an overall aim — such as caring for the health of their patients. It may seem bland and pointless to state the obvious, but unless there is some 'mission statement' the point of the team activities may be forgotten in the pursuit of details. Again, the members of the team will each have a different role within it. Consider the following case.

A 65-year-old man, who two months ago had a stroke, has returned to the hospital for a follow-up visit. He has made good progress and is now mobile, but still has a slight speech defect. During his initial admission he was noted to be hypertensive, and was started on drug treatment for this, and was put on a weight-reducing diet. He asks the following questions:
Will my treatment be changed today?
Do I need to continue with my speech therapy and physiotherapy?
Can I have a home help?
Should I continue with my diet?

It is obvious from a consideration of the questions that working in teams means being able to recognize one's own limitations and the strengths of others. Too strict a definition of roles, however, may set limitations for the team. Sometimes a centre forward has to play full back. It is necessary, however, if teams are to function properly, that members are able to practise together, and become aware of each other's strengths and weaknesses and share problems. There are interesting questions arising here, which we shall not discuss, about whether the doctor is always the appropriate team leader.

Finally, communication problems are important in teams. It is easy to think of communication as being patient-directed; but there is also the problem of communication within teams. This is a particularly common type of problem. One member of the team has made a decision, and perhaps even discussed it with the patient, but has not communicated it to the rest of the team. Often it is the junior nurse or doctor who is face-to-face with the patient asking the awkward or sensitive question. Unless each member of the team is involved then responses cannot be appropriate. We are here assuming that a decision has been made but not communicated within the team. There is, however, the other side of the coin — sometimes no decision has been made. Once again, confronted by a patient, what does the doctor or nurse do if a question is asked? This is a special problem when it has been decided (for good or ill) that a patient should not be told of the diagnosis. It may be that others in the team feel that this is not the way to proceed, and wish the patient to be informed. Situations of this kind lead to moral conflicts in teams, and we shall return to these when we consider ethics in medical education in Chapter 7.

3.8 Conclusions

1. There are three linked aspects to being a doctor: the aim, the role, and the skills; and it is important for an adequate account of the concept of a doctor that all three should be discussed.

2. In discussing the aims of medicine it is helpful to distinguish the *personal* aims a doctor might hope to fulfil through medical practice from both the *intrinsic* aims of medicine as such, and its *extrinsic* aims — those which can be fulfilled as a result of medical skills or knowledge.

3. The intrinsic aim of medicine is the pursuit of health narrowly conceived, although medical education may also assist doctors to pursue wider community health aims.

4. Doctors act in roles understood in terms of institutional rights and duties which give support of many kinds to both doctor and patient.

5. Medical skills derive from the intrinsic aim of medicine, but it is important to remember that health care is now delivered by teams.

6. Dr D in the opening vignette is worried about widening his scope to include what we are calling the extrinsic aims of medicine, whereas Dr S is too ambitious for the scope of medicine. Mr F lacks the communication skills which medical education should cultivate, and Dr I's education has not stressed the importance of teamwork.

Bibliography

Downie, R. S., Fyfe, Carol, and Tannahill, Andrew (1990). *Health promotion: models and values.* Oxford University Press.
Doxiadis, S. (ed.) (1990). *Ethics in health education.* Wiley, Chichester.

4 Education, training, and ethos

4.1 Some cases

4.1.1

Mr X is a student studying History at a university. He had excellent all-round qualifications and went up to university with several of his friends who entered the Medical Faculty. For the first few weeks he met his friends at lunch-time. But he now finds that they are much less interested in meeting him, and they are surrounded by friends from the Medical Faculty. Mr X was of the opinion that they were all students together who could compare notes and discuss their classes as they had previously done. But he now finds that whereas he is just a student they are medical students. Mr X finds them condescending and smug.

4.1.2

Dr J's wife has just left him. She points out that he works all the time and when he arrives (late) for meals he talks only about his patients or (and this is worse) his committees. When (rarely) they go to parties or out to dinner the other guests always seem to be doctors and their wives. Dr J doesn't see what he has done wrong. His view is that medicine is not like any old job; it involves 24-hours-per-day commitment to patients.

4.2 Does the doctor need to be educated?

This question is, in part, the modern version of an ancient dispute: is the doctor really a gentleman? Being a gentleman was mostly a matter of social status, but linked with this were implications for the type of education appropriate to a gentleman ('classical' or 'liberal') as opposed to that appropriate to a tradesman ('apprenticeship' or 'training'). In yet another sense the issue has been perpetuated in some respects by a division between theoretical and practical studies.

Before the nineteenth century brought its changes in medical education, the division between theory and practice was virtually complete: physicians knew the theory, and the others did the practice (sometimes under the physician's direction). The physicians were essentially literary men of broad culture and disdainful of 'manual labour' — which was left to healers of lower status. However, it was not just status which determined the type of education: this was also related to the doctor's role in society. Even today the question is appropriate: should we expect the doctor simply to be an 'expert' in the techniques of healing, or should doctors have a broader kind of capacity such that they might be expected to take an interest in matters outside their strictly professional range? Should the doctor be 'wise' in the way that a priest should be wise, or should the doctor be skilled in the way that an accountant should be skilled? Is there, or should there be, such a thing as a distinctively medical 'world-view', a humanity of medicine?

There is no doubt about the public's answer to this question: the doctor should be both wise and skilled; should be both educated and an expert. This demand seems to flow from the difficulty of discriminating between the strictly technical aspects of medicine and its moral or ethical outlook. It is also related to the reason why medicine is a paradigm 'profession'; a recognition of the vulnerability of the laity in the face of the competitive and commercial pressures of an unregulated market-place. We can therefore conclude that there is a powerful public expectation that the doctor should be educated as well as skilled; in other words, that the doctor's general competence should extend beyond the strictly vocational skills we would expect from a craftsman or expert. Several questions then arise concerning the extent to which this goal is being achieved, how it might be better achieved, or even whether it is a reasonable goal at all; perhaps the public should be led to expect less.

4.3   Some historical considerations

As we have already described, medicine was not always the unified profession which we see today. And the history of medicine tells us of two extreme and opposite tendencies of medical education: the physician, who was liberally educated but not trained in practice, and the surgeon or apothecary, who was trained in medicine but not liberally educated. When the profession began to become unified during the nineteenth century there was extensive debate concerning the nature of the balance that should be struck between these two possibilities.

There were two routes to registration. The student was either expected to study at university for a degree in either medicine or (later) surgery (or, later still, both); or else to study at some combination of university, hospital, and extra-mural college and by apprenticeship for a qualification from one of the corporations (the colleges and societies of physicians, surgeons, and apothecaries).

If we consider the situation which prevailed from the foundation of universities in the Middle Ages we find that the student physician was supposed to be an arts 'postgraduate': the schools of medicine (with those of theology and law) were 'higher' studies, to be undertaken only after the common arts curriculum had been completed to MA standard. Thus the MD was a higher doctorate akin to the DD (doctor of divinity) and LL D (doctor of laws). Throughout much of the nineteenth century, although the requirement for an MA was dropped, there was an attempt to enforce a requirement for initial university arts study preliminary to medicine. For example, the Newcastle School of Medicine required previous residence at Durham University for a year of full-time arts if the medical degree was to be taken. However, the requirements were generally ineffective, and students simply bypassed the degree by taking the Apothecaries' and/or Surgeons' qualifications; so that eventually this stipulation was dropped in favour of 'evidence' of previous study of the arts.

The case of Newcastle shows in microcosm what happened generally: that the liberal study considered necessary for 'education' in medicine was excluded from the university curriculum and converted into part of a preliminary or qualifying examination which was prepared for extra-murally — usually at school. We thus reach the present situation, where what was once a preliminary MA has been eroded to the sixteen-plus examination passes (principally English, mathematics, and a foreign language) which are necessary for matriculation. There was also a prolonged, although unsuccessful, rearguard action to insist upon a similar preliminary study of Latin (duplicating the ineffective attempt to insist upon preliminary Greek during the nineteenth century); but the special status of Classics could not be convincingly defended. In such respects medicine reflected the widespread breakdown of consensus throughout educated society as to what defined the core of a 'cultured' education.

Our discussion leaves to one side the question of whether university study centred around Classics (at Oxford), mathematics (at Cambridge), or moral philosophy (in the ancient Scottish universities) really had the educative effect of the kind aimed for and claimed on their behalf (although there is strong evidence that, taken in the cultural context of the time in Scotland, moral philosophy probably did). What is clear is that in the past there was a serious attempt to ensure that the doctor was liberally educated, while at present there is not. This change in purpose went hand-in-hand with the universities taking over from the corporations the role of providing a licence to practise medicine (although there are still vestiges of the old system in the alternative qualifications of the London 'conjoint' and LMSSA, and the Scottish 'triple'). What seems to have happened, more by chance than design, is that the universities have in the end adopted for their qualifications the goals of the medical corporations of early Victorian times: in taking over licensing the universities would seem to have taken over the ethos appropriate for apprenticeship and training. The ideal of a liberally educated doctor has been lost: if students are not liberally educated when they come up to university, then there is nothing in the curriculum to encourage them to be liberally educated from that point onwards. So much for the liberal ideal. That battle may seem to have been fought and lost.

It should be noted, however, that the widespread emergence of 'medical humanities' in medical schools of the USA, and the beginnings of such a movement in the UK, are perhaps evidence of a resurgence of the liberal ideal. We shall discuss a place for the arts in Chapter 7. But the story of the 'extra-vocational' education does not end there, because if there has been a progressive decline at least until recently in the role of 'the arts' in the education of a doctor, there has been a reciprocal rise in the role of science. This emergence of an ideal of scientific education has gathered strength as the arts have declined.

The 'science take-over' of the medical curriculum gathered force during late Victorian times in response to progress in medical research. In part this had a strictly vocational goal, the aim being to increase understanding of the body (and later mind) in health and disease, so that clinical practice might be improved. But in addition to this the idea grew that the study of science might have an 'intrinsic' value analogous to the 'intrinsic' value of the arts (and might therefore be educationally superior to the arts, since it had both vocational relevance *and* general educative potential). In this view, a scientific education teaches a range of skills and attitudes which are generally applicable to broad aspects of life — medical practice in particular. The specific science is of only secondary importance, as all true sciences are assumed to share these educative elements. This is the reason given for inclusion of scientific information in the curriculum beyond what is required for clinical practice, and also for giving support to intercalated science degrees in medicine.

As we shall argue in one of the chapters concerning the preclinical curriculum, however (Chapter 6), the way in which science is actually taught leaves much to be desired. In particular, its educational potential is strictly limited by its mode of presentation, while the claims for its vocational relevance are over-emphasized. If the universities were serious about using science as the route to a general education then they would have to set about it in a rather different fashion than is done at present. Let us go on to consider the contrast between science (or any other subject) taught as part of 'education' and taught as part of 'training'.

4.4 Education and training

The philosophy of education since 1960 has been greatly influenced by the many writings of R. S. Peters, and it may be helpful to begin by looking at the distinctions which he drew between education and training. It should be said that he developed the distinctions in slightly different ways in various works, and that what we offer here is a paraphrase of his distinctions rather than an exposition of any one way in which he drew them. He argues that there are three main criteria which an activity must satisfy if it is to be called 'education'.

The most important criterion is that something worthwhile or valuable for its own sake must be passed on in any activity which is properly to be called education. It is obvious that Fagan's class in picking pockets in Dicken's *Oliver Twist*, while it may be training, is not education, because it is actually harmful. There are also neutral activities which may count as 'training' but are not 'education' in terms of Peters's distinction. For example, a student can be trained to give an intravenous injection; but this is not 'education', even although it is used to help a patient. Again, the study of medicine more generally is obviously related to the provision of the trained manpower needed by the health service; but this end-result is not what makes medicine an educational activity. Rather, it is the intrinsic value of the human biology and behavioural sciences essential to the study of medicine which makes it an educational activity, for they provide ways of understanding the world and making sense of experience which are worth while in themselves, regardless of the practical uses to which this understanding may be put. To the extent that we concentrate on the practical uses of medicine we are thinking of it as 'training' for a further end, and to the extent that we see it as a way of understanding the complexities of the human body and behaviour we are thinking of it as education.

The second criterion which any activity must satisfy if it is to be educational is that it must have a wide perspective. Thus, activities such as science, history, literature, and so on are central to education not only because they are valuable in themselves but also because they may widen and deepen one's understanding of many other matters. For example, imagine a historian of the French Revolution who was surprised when he was told that a study of this period led people to think of such matters as social justice, and said that he was just interested in the 'the facts'. Or, to use a medical example, consider the oncologist who cannot understand why her subject should be of interest to plant biologists or molecular geneticists, as she is only interested in 'treating cancer'. It might be more appropriate to say that such a person had been trained as a historian or oncologist than that he or she had been educated. A person may be trained in circumscribed skills; but we reserve the term 'education' for activities which broaden and deepen our understanding.

The third condition which any educational activity must satisfy, besides being valuable in itself and related to other activities thought valuable, is that those who are engaged in it must come to care about what they are doing. Suppose that students have completed a university course in biology, or chemistry (activities which are valuable in themselves and have a wide perspective) but thereafter show no interest in these subjects. We might say that they have been highly trained, but if they do not care about what they know they are not educated.

To these central criteria we can add others, some of which are mentioned by Peters himself in various writings. Fourthly, education implies that a person's whole outlook has been transformed — it involves 'wholeness'; whereas training suggests a competence of more limited scope.

Fifthly, training may sometimes actually involve a narrowing of the consciousness to master certain techniques. An example of this might be specialized surgical procedures requiring a great deal of expertise which can only come from practice and experience. Education, on the other hand, has to do with opening out, with 'educing', which releasing and liberating (as Rita found in the film and play *Educating Rita*).

Sixthly, it follows from (4) and (5) that the educator must employ different methods from those of the trainer. The educator must always employ morally acceptable, person-respecting methods. For example, to teach by fear, indoctrination, coercion, or hidden persuasion is not to educate, but it can be to train. Again, education encourages critical thought, and must be a two-way process; whereas training can be based on imitation or even on parroting.

4.5   Applications and implications for medicine: some models

It would undoubtedly be possible to develop the distinctions between these concepts even further; but perhaps enough has been said to enable us to distinguish the two. Let us now provisionally accept these distinctions, and apply them to the activities which go on in medical schools and universities. A number of models may be developed which highlight the differences described above.

As a first bracketing shot at application we might say that whereas faculties of arts at least attempt to engage in

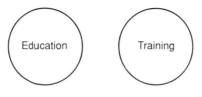

Fig. 4.1

educational activities, faculties of law and medicine attempt to engage in training. This shot is not wildly inaccurate, as can be seen from the following common situation. The proud possessor of first-class honours in English may be disconcerted at his graduation ceremony when his friend who is graduating in medicine asks him: 'What's your degree in English for?' No one will ever ask the medical graduate that question. The arts graduate may be able to say that as a result of his degree he is being taken on as a graduate trainee in an industry; but that is not what the degree was for. It was not for anything beyond itself; whereas the subjects studied in medicine are studied for a purpose — to train the student to treat the sick. Indeed, even the methods of teaching in medicine typically fit the training paradigm: a large amount of rote learning examined by multiple-choice examinations. If we accept the distinction between education and training outlined above, and also the application of it to medical studies, we are left with the simple relationship (Fig. 4.1) that education and training are seen as separate activities, training being more appropriate in medicine.

Two lines of criticism of this oversimplified scheme might be pursued, a less and a more radical line. The less radical criticism reminds us that educational as well as training activities take place in medicine. Thus, a course in medical statistics or clinical physics, for example, may be taught, received, and examined in the mode of training, for the good reason that typical medical students do not have the sort of mathematical background or the sort of interests to make these subjects educational for them. Their teachers may also have a hearty contempt for the 'service course' they are providing. But it is also possible that a well-taught course in biochemistry, for example, may satisfy the criteria for an educational rather than

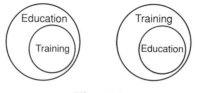

Fig. 4.2

a training activity. It can be taught in a way which encourages a critical understanding of bodily processes, as a subject worthwhile for its own sake, as one which suggests linkages with wider systems of biological and chemical knowledge, and as one which students might come to care about and follow up on their own during the period of continuing education. The result of studying courses in this way is that they have a value of their own independent of their use. In other words, they are educational activities. Accepting this (less radical) criticism of the initial distinction we have the scheme shown in Fig. 4.2, depending on the emphases.

Let us now challenge the distinction on a more radical basis. First, the 'training' initially outlined is a narrowly conceived type of training, as in trade, whereas the 'education' described is a broadly conceived concept of one sort of education, often called liberal education. But this is not a fair contrast; training can be broad-based, as in training for the ministry of the Church. Secondly, the contrast between the concepts builds in an alleged difference in the point of each: education is assumed to be aimed at the growth or reconstruction of the understanding (an aim intrinsic to the activity) whereas training is assumed to be aimed at an operative efficiency (an extrinsic aim). But the concepts are in some respects closer than that contrast suggests, since acquiring an operative efficiency may be a necessary part of coming to understand, while, conversely, operative efficiency may not be possible without understanding. For example, having been trained in some biochemical procedure may be a precondition of successfully understanding some more advanced topic such as diabetes in pregnancy, while a precondition of being successfully trained to cure people of some affliction may be an understanding of the life

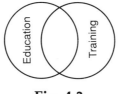

Fig. 4.3

cycle of a certain parasite. Thirdly, it seems a doubtful point that education properly speaking has no aim beyond itself. That may be true of one kind of education — liberal education; but it does not seem to be true of the concept as a whole, and it is not helpful to allow the narrower idea of liberal education to hijack the concept. The many specific forms of education, such as health education, management education, and medical education, obviously have further aims; but since they also have wide knowledge-bases and cognitive perspectives, and can be taught and learned in a caring way, they can also be seen as valuable for their own sakes. We therefore propose that preparing students to be doctors is both a training activity and an educational activity, and should be seen as shown in Fig. 4.3.

A further point is that education should be transmitted in a morally acceptable way, and that indoctrination is unacceptable (see criterion 6, above). Yet in medicine a great deal of indoctrination occurs. The 'hidden agenda' in medicine, and the transmission of values and beliefs, occur in this manner, and may be very necessary in the maintenance of standards. If 'indoctrination' is considered too strong a word for the process we could substitute terms such as 'initiation' or 'professionalization'. But, whatever the most appropriate terms, there is and ought to be a process of nurture through which learners assimilate the value base of medicine. While this may be subrational, and cannot therefore be included in Peters's criteria, it is of the first importance to the educated doctor. Let us now look at this important issue in more detail.

4.6 Ethos and professionalization

One subject about which both the most conservative doctors and their most radical critics agree, is that there is a particular 'world-view' associated with the practice of medicine: it is this we will call the morality of medicine. (Medical morality should not be confused with the field of 'medical ethics' — the study of specifically ethical dimensions of medical practice — although the two subjects are intimately linked. We are using 'morality' in an older and more general sense.)

Before we discuss whether or not this medical morality is a 'good thing' it will be worth discussing just what it might be. Of course, when we are considering tens of thousands of individuals from a fairly wide background we will find a considerable variety of world-views; but nevertheless there is also homogeneity. Firstly, the medical morality is a practical morality, by which we mean that it is directed towards action. This would seem to derive from the constraints of clinical practice, in which a decision must always be made, even if that decision is to postpone the decision.

This shows in the medical view of science. For a doctor, science is a goal-directed activity, and the direction is towards improved clinical practice. In contrast, the scientist is regulated by goals *internal* to science itself (this is what is meant by science 'for its own sake'). It also shows in medical impatience with speculation of all kinds: indeed a 'short attention span', sometimes showing itself as a hard-headed approach, is often a fault of clinicians — although it is a 'fault' which has the benefits of efficiency and productivity in clinical practice.

'Decision' is a key word in our discussion, because it is also characteristic of doctors to be decisive. When the caricature doctor is at fault it is more often for deciding too soon (without sufficient consideration of evidence) than too late: at any rate doctors do not usually experience much psychological difficulty about making up their minds. Such resolution contrasts with the attitudes of some other professions — and is one explanation of why doctors tend to adopt a dominant role in committees!

There are many other features of the medical world-view. For example, it is most characteristically associated with clinical practice: with the face-to-face involvement with patients. And linked with this there is the practical orientation: doctors are concerned with disease, with illness, with the breakdown of normal function. The doctor *qua* doctor does not have much to say about healthy, 'normal' human existence, although the doctor as a person may do — this is part of what we called the extrinsic aim of medicine.

Perhaps enough has been sketched to conclude that there is something we can call a medical world-view. If so, one striking feature is that it has a great deal to do with the nature of medicine as a profession. To put it another way, medicine is characterized by a high level of collegiality or solidarity. This is a great source of strength, as well as a possible source of harm, as when in the face of any criticism there is a tendency for doctors always to stick together. We can now proceed to examine, in a sociological fashion, how medical education is involved in the process of producing the medical morality.

One part is the evolution of an *espirit de corps*. The military metaphor is appropriate in emphasizing that such a spirit is morally neutral in itself, and can as easily be directed to the business of killing people as healing them. Various factors combine to produce *esprit de corps* within the medical school. Firstly, the students are divided into classes (often large) each of which is treated as a unit, and the classes are all taught together in big lectures and practical sessions whenever this is possible. Furthermore, all the students in the same class share a curriculum which is broadly, and sometimes exactly, the same as those of the other class-members. Such features are common to many medical schools during the preclinical period. The sheer bulk of information may forcibly impose the subject on the minds of the undergraduates. To some extent the medical students are usually physically set apart from other undergraduates in a medical school or college. And commonly curricular activities are reinforced by informal student societies. Such factors may play a greater or lesser role in inculcating a sense of loyalty, tradition, or whatever it might be called, even in the earliest years; an attitude which becomes directed partly at the institution and its members, but also towards medicine itself.

In the clinical years the process gathers momentum: the university terms are longer and vacations shorter; a standard of quasi-professional behaviour and dress is encouraged; 'out of hours' study is increasingly expected. Some factors are established explicitly, by lecture or textbook; but most of the medical morality comes from apprenticeship, from the learning process described as 'modelling', whereby the acolyte becomes identified with the 'master' across a whole range of interlinking behaviours, attitudes, and emotions. This is the time during which the beginnings of a 'bedside manner'; are adopted, and ways of relating to patients, other health care workers, and the public are internalized. This induction may be very enjoyable; and it is usual that the clinical years at medical school are the time of the greatest idealism concerning the values of a medical way of life.

Following qualification, the years spent as a junior hospital doctor present a challenge to the idealism of student life, as these values are tested against the rigours of round-the-clock practice at the bottom of a hierarchy. The result may be cynicism and/or disillusionment (common among junior doctors); but anti-professional behaviour is kept within fairly strict boundaries by the already-established medical morality, and also by the hierarchical system of job appointments based on references and recommendations from senior staff. It is easier to externalize discontent by projecting it on to the patients (or nurses) than by challenging the medical profession. The solidarity of the medical profession acts as a powerful support through the rigours of these years, and in conditions of overwork and inexperience it is reassuring to know that, if or when things go wrong, then your colleagues will back you up — that the doctors will stick together (at least in public).

The fact of professional solidarity is a double-edged weapon — it was characterized by Bernard Shaw as a 'conspiracy against the laity'; but its benefits should not be underestimated. In the first place, medicine is intrinsically an unpleasant job, in the sense that it involves contact with blood, sweat, and tears (and worse); but, more seriously, it involves life-and-death decisions and actions. All of which means that a mistake may have consequences of the utmost seriousness — and everybody makes mistakes. It is of the greatest importance that, on the one hand, mistakes can be acknowledged and corrected; and, on the other hand, that the junior doctor is supported through the mistakes to develop the highest level of skill (because if 'everybody makes mistakes' then this applies particularly to the inexperienced new recruit).

Ideally, the profession offers a protected environment within which mistakes can be admitted and transcended without the potentially arbitrary and destructive effect of uninformed public appraisal. What is more, the relative independence of the professional ethos is a powerful source of resistance to potentially damaging external pressures. The concerted nature of BMA campaigns against government proposals to commercialize and politicize the National Health Service came as something of a surprise to politicians and the public. The campaign did not mainly stress doctors' financial self-interest, but rather what was considered to be the 'general interest'. It is worth noting that such qualified altruism is only made possible by the economic fact that doctors are relatively insulated from the whiplash of the market-place, and given guarantees of an assured livelihood. This fact could, of course, be unilaterally broken by a government's removing the medical profession's monopoly and its peculiar privileges and protections.

So, how does medical morality compare with other types of professional-group morality, such as those of lawyers, priests, or teachers? One immediately striking difference is that medical morality commands a broad measure of public support, as opposed to that of lawyers, who are regarded as self-seeking; priests, who are regarded as well-meaning but misguided; and teachers, who are blamed for everything. Comparing medical morality with the *public* morality — the mood of the nation or 'popular opinion' — we might say that the latter is deeply fragmented and unstable, and increasingly susceptible to manipulation by political, commercial, and media forces (last week a campaign against homelessness, this week the horror of social security 'scroungers', and next week child abuse — or maybe the right of parents instead).

In such entropic conditions the existence of a stable and solid system of morality becomes even more valuable. This seems to be acknowledged by the public deference to medical morality. This deference is compatible with powerful criticism of individual doctors or even the health service; indeed these criticism are often made in terms of failing to live up to the standards of good medical morals. In a situation of short-termism and crass exploitation within the public domain, there is an important place for the integrated medical world-view.

This, however, is not the whole story, because medical morality is not the whole story. Medical morality is, as we have

already stated, inevitably incomplete: it is concerned only with
certain limited aspects of life — with illness and disease. The
combination of medical solidarity with the fragmentation of
public discourse can allow medicine to overstep its bounds — it
can lead to a lack of perspective. If medical morality is to function properly it must be placed within the scheme of society
as a whole — its limits defined, its relationship to other
world-views made clear. It is not satisfactory that the medical
viewpoint should simply take over all other viewpoints by
default, that the problems of life should all be medicalized. So
that while we support strongly the existence of what we have
called medical morality, we must also emphasize that this will
be a good thing only if it is taken in perspective. Doctors,
through a combination of excessive busyness and solidarity,
can easily lose their broad perspectives to become not just
workaholic, but blinkered to the point of not knowing *when* to
use their medical skill — although they might know very well
how. This is often said to be the characteristic sin of the surgeon
— yet it applies across a much wider spread of the profession.
And it is exactly here that the university part of medical
education can make its most valuable contribution.

What seems to be needed is for doctors to be encouraged in a
countervailing world-view, against which the medical morality
may be contrasted and tested. It is for just this reason that we
have placed emphasis on the importance of the doctor's being
an *educated* person, and not only a skilled one. We have suggested a training in science as one candidate for a countervailing (and intrinsically critical) discipline: but the social
sciences, humanities, and arts and crafts are also suitable for
this purpose, and can, as we shall show, be justified as part of a
medical curriculum. None of these would necessarily make a
more effective doctor, by narrow clinical audit criteria; but they
would encourage, so far as is possible, wisdom in medicine.

Education might also encourage a more appropriate degree
of responsiveness to the needs of the public. Whereas it may be
a good thing that medicine does not turn with public opinion
like a weather-vane, it is a bad thing when stable and legitimate
public desires for such things as humane antenatal check-ups,
unhurried consultations, or continuity of care in hospital out-
patients' departments can be completely ignored and disregarded

despite years of agitation. The social sciences and humanities can help with this kind of responsiveness, as we shall argue later in Chapter 7.

What are needed are: an antidote to medical arrogance which does not dilute medical strength; the introduction of alternative perspectives against which the medical morality may be contrasted and through which improvements may result; and a critical and corrective mechanism whereby knowledge and practice do not ossify into unchallengable dogma. We stress that medical morality is an immensely valuable resource, not just for medicine, but for society at large. What is required is not, therefore, destruction of that professional solidarity which generates and sustains the rational moral system, but expansion and completion of this morality by a process of education.

4.7 Conclusions

1. Medical knowledge changes and develops, and the doctor must have an open and flexible mind to receive new ideas. Openness and flexibility are features of the educated rather than the narrowly trained mind.

2. The understanding that is part of education has standards built into it. Awareness of intellectual standards is of the first importance for diagnosis and treatment of patients.

3. The appreciation of activities valuable for their own sakes, such as science, can provide a lifelong interest which is one safeguard against the despair and disillusionment of much medical practice.

4. Caring for a subject is analogous to caring for a person: it is the ethical dimension of the educational. Doctors have a responsibility to become involved in continuing education and training if the best patient-care is to be the prime objective. They will fulfil this responsibility more willingly and adequately if they also care for their subject.

5. Educated doctors, as distinct from trained technicians, have appropriate professional attitudes. These are acquired through a process of unconscious assimilation, or from contagion with seniors who have the appropriate attitude. In 4.1.1 Mr X, the History student, is coming up against the fact that his former friends are beginning the process of initiation or professionalization; he may just need to recognize this. The problem with Dr J in 4.1.2 is that he has not recovered from this process. He has drowned in the medical ethos, and requires resuscitation with some strong countervailing culture.

Bibliography

Calman, K. C. and Downie, R. S. (1988) Education and training in medicine. *Medical Education*, **22**, 488–91.

Peters, R. S. (1966). *Ethics and education*. Allen and Unwin, London.

Turner, G. G. and Arnison, W. D. (1934). *The Newcastle upon Tyne School of Medicine 1834–1934*. Andrew Reid & Co., Newcastle.

Youngson, A. J. (1989). Medical education in the later 19th century: the science take-over. *Medical Education*, **23**, 490–1.

Part II: Practice

5 *Selection for medicine*

5.1 A case

Dr A is the Admissions Officer to a Medical Faculty. As usual the limited number of places available have been greatly oversubscribed with applications. The Admissions Committee, after a long meeting, decided that he was to be flexible in his admission policy, so he analyses the applications, and finds the following. The majority of applicants have applied straight from school, and have excellent scientific qualifications. It would indeed be possible to fill all the places with these applicants (and this has been Dr A's previous practice). Dr A also notes a number with less good scientific qualifications, but all-round intellectual interests (in previous years he might have rejected these). There are others again who have less than first-rate qualifications (although as good as Dr A achieved many years earlier), but who have done well at sport. He remembers that some older doctors favour such applicants. He also has several miscellaneous candidates, including one nurse and several graduates in the 'Humanities'. All the applicants in this category are older, and their scientific qualifications are relatively weak. How should Dr A choose? How can he defend his choice? The Committee told him he should speak to the candidates if he is in doubt; but Dr A is not entirely sure what he would be looking for in an interview.

5.2 The best students

Selection is of key importance to medical education. What sort of students are recruited at the beginning is a major determinant of what kind of doctors come out at the end. Many aspects of intellectual capacity and personality are already well-established before children reach university age, so that education is inevitably constrained by the nature of the people involved. That much is uncontroversial, but emphasizes the extent to which the whole of medical education — as discussed at length in this book — operates within guidelines dictated by this first stage, preliminary to the actual education itself.

When it comes to selecting students for medical school, we are faced with a number of distinct possibilities — some of which may be mutually exclusive. Should it be the purpose of selection to choose those people who will best be able to complete the undergraduate medical training — those who will score most highly in examinations? Or perhaps a longer perspective is preferable; to choose those who will make the best *doctors* — whatever that means? Or, alternatively — and acknowledging that in many ways medicine is a *privileged* job — should we ensure that a proportion of the available places should be awarded to specific kinds of 'deserving' people (women, perhaps, or poor people?) — so that it does not remain a middle-class male preserve? Should the acceptance of students to study medicine perhaps be seen in an even wider perspective, in terms of the whole population of university students, and what they 'ought' to be studying in terms of the 'needs' of the nation?

On top of all this, there is the vexed question of *how* to select students. What are the essential preliminary subjects (A-levels or Scottish Highers) and standards; should there be interviews, and, if so, what form should they take; what value is it reasonable to place on the head teacher's report or its equivalent? We will examine these questions in turn.

In a very real sense, there is *no* problem in selecting medical students. However things may have been in the past, for the last couple of decades and more there has been a glut of good candidates for medical school; the entrance examination requirements are currently higher (a measure of demand from highly academic pupils) than for any other major subject except veterinary medicine. The very title of this chapter gives away the point; we talk in terms of *selection*, and have no worries about attracting enough students in the first place. By the usual 'academic' standards, then, there is no problem, and medical school places can simply be 'rationed' by raising entrance requirements until they balance the demand. It is not absolutely necessary to take our enquiry any further if we are happy with this situation. After all, high academic qualifications in the students might be presumed to reflect a high general ability; and it is uncontroversial that, at the extremes, a group of students with a strong academic background will outperform a group with a weak background — by a wide range of professional criteria. Recruitment of 'star' school pupils brings prestige to an institution, and this prestige then attracts more of the 'best' pupils, forcing up academic standards in a positive-feedback cycle of increasing status. However, even (or especially) in those universities most famous for high entrance requirements, we will find the view that there is much more to selection than this: that there is an effort to choose well-rounded, or balanced, personalities — and that this is even more important in the case of medicine.

The literature is full of papers (too many to list) looking for correlations between achievements at school and at university or after — analysing, for example, performance at various school subjects at O- or A-level to find the best guide to success at second MB or final examinations or beyond. The results are very variable between studies (some claim O-levels as the best predictors, others A-levels; some say biology is the optimum guide, others chemistry). However, correlations are never so tight as to be absolutely compelling. Indeed, the major conclusion must be that predictions are so vague as to encourage a greater level of experimentation than at present.

Even if this question were to be settled unambiguously — with results applicable across all medical schools and in all countries — it would still not tell us which school subjects *should* be preliminary. The current consensus would seem to be that a general academic education to the age of sixteen, followed by a more-or-less general scientific education for the next year or two, is what is required. The inclusion of mathematics and/or physics is justified more on their reputation as 'hard' sciences with implications of intellectual rigour than on their vocational relevance.

Other critics of what they see as medical narrowness of attitude would favour a 'humane' school education, with the vocational science being done at university (we shall argue (Chapter 7) that there may, alternatively, be a place for humane education actually within the medical school). It is at this point that the discussion spills over into considering 'what makes a good doctor'. (See Chapter 11 for further discussion of this complex topic.)

As for *how* best to select students the answer is quite simple: we do not know. The present system is a combination of (mostly) written examinations and a recommendation from an academic such the head teacher. This may or may not be supplemented by an interview. About interviews, it is sufficient to say that they are known to be of very limited reliability and validity, and prone to distortion by prejudice and snap-judgements. Their value seems to be mainly to reassure the institution and the applicant that things are being done properly.

Overall, though, the problem of finding medical students who are competent to complete the course successfully is another non-problem. Medical students are good enough to do this already: indeed, it might be said that they are too good. The admissions hurdle is so high (and the failure rate so low) that there is no selecting left for the university to do. In other words, people are selected to become doctors at the time they are selected for medical school: if you are accepted as a medical student you have been virtually accepted into the medical profession, and you will become a doctor.

One alternative, which is practised in some other countries, is to admit many more students initially than will qualify ultimately, and to fail a high proportion of them during the course: a so called 'open access' system. By this method the university does the selecting instead of the schools. However, while this gives more people the chance to become doctors, it does tend to result in poor-quality teaching due to the unmanageably vast numbers of students in the early years. Although late selection might, in theory, open the way to a more considered estimate of the good students, in practice the numbers force a reliance upon mass examination much as at school. Open access is also an expensive option in a situation where university education is subsidised by the state. It is probable that the money can be better spent than by giving a large number of students a year or two of inferior-quality study which most of them will inevitably fail.

5.3 Medicine in context

Such is the success of medical recruitment in terms of the students' academic ability that some authors have pointed out that this has been achieved at the price of standards in other subjects. In particular they mean the pure or applied sciences and engineering, where (broadly speaking) entrance requirements have had to be lowered as those in medicine have been raised. Furthermore, it is asserted that the job of being a doctor is not one which would necessarily appeal to a person of a seriously intellectual bent; or, more importantly, that it might be a job which would be done *better* by someone of a practical and friendly disposition: the opposite of the types selected for by academic high-jumps.

The upshot of this kind of view would be that selection by academic criteria should not go beyond the minimum necessary to complete the course successfully; and that, after this has been achieved, no advantage should attach to yet higher grades. Or, more moderately, that while high grades might carry a statistical advantage, places should also be set aside for students with lower qualifications and, presumably, more appropriate character traits. By such means medicine would voluntarily relinquish its grip on the high-flying scientific schoolchildren, and liberate more for other subjects where (a) they would meet more intellectual challenges or (b) they would be more useful to the community.

The phrase 'more appropriate character traits' requires further comment. It has been suggested that the appropriate behaviour patterns for *most* doctors should perhaps be rather less glamorous than at present: that the emphasis should be placed on a character of stability, warmth, reliability, kindliness, modesty, and a blend of gently sceptical conservatism with a responsible attitude to maintaining professional competence. Such traits may be more often seen in those with less theoretical and scholarly aptitudes than the students selected at present. One way to increase the proportion of such doctors might be to select students in their twenties, when the personality has had time to develop and prove itself in life, rather than at the age of seventeen or eighteen, when future character is uncertain. Needless to say, selection of 'mature' students would not, of itself, produce a different personality type if — as at present — they continue to be chosen only on the basis of their academic record (upper second class honours degree or better).

Such ideas are looking beyond undergraduate success, and towards a lifetime of medicine. As such they suffer from the uncertainties about what constitutes a good doctor *now*; but what is even more uncertain is what will constitute a good doctor in five, ten, or twenty years time! It is unsurprising that the medical schools choose to emphasize the relative predict-ability of undergraduate performance as opposed to long-term professional competence. Nevertheless, the two aims must be balanced.

Eccentric as the above ideas may seem, they put the claims of medicine into a broad context, and force us to think about the kinds of qualities which we would wish prospective doctors to exhibit. And they make us ask whether we would prefer a homogeneous intake (of school-leaving-age academic high flyers) or whether some provision should be made deliberately to select across a variety of aptitudes, ages, and personality types.

5.4   Medicine as a privilege

The fact, already commented on, that we have no difficulty in attracting large numbers of able students to apply for medicine deserves further comment. What accounts for this buoyant demand? If we leave aside the considerable attractions of a life in medicine, one important factor is *security*. A degree in medi-cine is widely received as an entry into a secure livelihood; as secure as any other possible job, at any rate. How, then, has such security been obtained? Medicine was not always thus: throughout much of history there have been considerable periods when it was exceedingly difficult to make a living by practising as a doctor.

The answer is that medical graduates have a monopoly over the vital areas of health care (N.H.S. jobs, prescribing, etc.), and that access to this medical monopoly is strictly regulated. The numbers of doctors are limited to such an extent that they are all (virtually) guaranteed a secure livelihood and a reasonable standard of living. Of course, there is much more to it than this; 'demand' for medical services is not fixed, salaries are not determined only by scarcity value, and so on. But, at the end of the day, the medical profession has been able to obtain for itself a remarkable degree of long-term security; and this is based upon a strictly regulated entry.

It is worth reiterating that this was not always the case. Until late Victorian times there was not sufficient money to go around all the qualified doctors, mostly because there was no regulation of the numbers of practitioners. Or, to put it another way; the number of people entering medicine was dictated by their perception of whether they could make a good living after they had qualified (not least, to pay off the debts incurred during training). The numbers of doctors were limited only by the numbers of training positions (mostly apprenticeships), themselves limited by the numbers of people who could afford them. Doctors were in competition with each other to an extent which is strange to us today: fierce competition encouraged not only positive measures, such as obtaining more and better qualifications or recommendations, but also *negative* measures, such as discrediting the opposition! It is the fear of this kind of situation — doctors at each other's throats and undermining each other's reputations — which lies behind today's powerful professional ethical code, whereby 'doctors always stick together', and never criticize a colleague.

This preamble is intended to establish that medical graduates have certain institutionalized privileges. It is possible to argue that this makes the business of selecting medical students for admission to this privileged group a matter of broad concern to society. For example, the fact that medicine is largely a middle-class preserve is worrying to some people (as is the 'dynastic' element in medicine — children of doctors being *perceived* to have a better chance of getting into medical school, although this is probably not really the case to any significant degree).

Of course, such considerations are not unique to medicine, but apply to every profession — indeed to many skilled trades, or to any situation where demand for traineeships exceeds their supply. The nature of this problem can be shown by analogy with law. Barristers and advocates have a professional monopoly of certain kinds of legal work which enables many of them to become extremely wealthy; furthermore judges are selected from among their ranks. On the one hand the *quality* of barristers seems to be high, and in this sense there is no problem about their methods of selection. On the other hand, both the nature of the professional training and the conditions in which novices must establish their practice ensure that advocacy is the virtual preserve of the upper middle classes (those with the ability to find a 'private income' for several years). Is this situation a cause for concern? Is it an example of entrenched privilege successfully defending its class interests? Or is it the price we pay, as a society, for an independent and highly professional legal system? The same kinds of questions apply to medicine, and impinge upon the selection of medical students. There may be other reasons for wishing to have a broader mix of social types in medicine. A greater diversity of background would tend to result in a more flexible profession, with a wider sympathy and sense of responsibility. However, we cannot ask too much. Medical school selectors have their work cut out simply trying to choose *the best* (by whatever criteria) students from those who apply, without trying to compensate for the inequalities of our socio-political system. If they try to make this compensation by positively discriminating in favour of disadvantaged students, in the first place this is not likely to be effective (in terms of society at large it will be mere drop in the ocean); in the second place it will result in students of a lower quality (and, presumably, doctors of a lower quality); and in the third place it will harm the institution itself by diluting or confusing its commitment to medical excellence.

This suggests that, while questions such as the balance between the factors of sex, class, race, religion, appearance, health status, regional background, or whatever are important, to the community at large, they should not be part of the remit of medical selection (except where there is evidence of discrimination and unfair prejudice). If, on consideration, it is felt that there is a problem, and that 'something must be done' to recruit more students from specific sectors of society, then this is a matter for the overall regulatory bodies, a matter of setting-out a compulsory framework applicable to all medical schools (a 'level pitch') before the admissions officers proceed to choose 'the best' from the group on offer.

In other words, 'affirmative action' must come from above — not from individual universities. A multitude of *ad hoc* policies implemented by miscellaneous admissions officers of various medical schools cannot be properly evaluated or criticized, and is open to considerable abuse. Selection itself is problematic enough, without trying to make it a panacea for the world's ills. If selectors are trying to do too much too well, they will end by failing to do anything properly.

All this involves a frank admission that — in selection — we do not know what we are doing, and an honest attempt at damage-limitation in the light of this incompetence. At present we might consider ways to avoid putting all our medical eggs into one personality basket!

5.5 Conclusions

1. There are several criteria for selection, some of them mutually exclusive; and even the individual criteria are far from straightforward.

2. In the face of uncertainty as to what is required, a deliberately eclectic approach to selection seems the wisest.

3. Medical schools should perhaps unashamedly adopt a policy of 'picking and mixing' the characters and aptitudes of their students — once they have fulfilled the necessary level of academic achievement.

Bibliography

Horrobin, D. M. (1978). *Medical hubris: a reply to Ivan Illich*. Churchill Livingstone, Edinburgh.

Louden, I. (1986). *Medical care and the general practitioner 1750–1850*. Oxford University Press.

McCormick, J. (1990). What is a good doctor? A personal view. *Family Practice*, **6**, 247–8.

Shuster, S. (1980) No career for academic high fliers. *British Medical Journal*, **280**, 335.

6 The preclinical curriculum: biological sciences

6.1 Some cases

It is commonly remarked that, whatever their differences in experience, it is hard to distinguish between doctors trained in different medical schools, even a few years after qualification. Whether or not this is true, it emphasizes the difficulty of finding correlations between educational events and subsequent professional practice. Lacking such information we are compelled to judge the educational value of the early years of medical school by rational, rather than by empirical, means. Such assessment is necessary because uncertainty about the scientific value of the preclinical curriculum is common. Consider the following cases.

6.1.1
Miss B is a second-year medical student. She has excellent scientific qualifications and some experience of voluntary work with the elderly. Miss B is depressed because her friends in Medicine study all the time (and she seems to be out of touch with her previous friends from school who take other subjects). She has been led to believe that her first few years would be hard because they would be very 'scientific'. She has found however that there is very little science, as distinct from endless learning of names. But there is so much of that, that she does not have time any more to visit the elderly people she used to look after. She has spoken to her adviser about withdrawing from Medicine, and the adviser assumed that this was because she was finding the course too difficult. Miss B wonders whether a course can at one and the same time be both much too time-consuming and much too undemanding.

6.1.2
Dr D entered medical school with high scientific qualifications. He found the course easy but time-consuming, and he did not especially enjoy his job in general practice ('Too many neurotic women and geriatrics.'). He was of the opinion that his career might develop if he were able to carry out some research. He submitted a research proposal concerned with the effect of hyperventilation on a range of disorders. To his annoyance the

research ethics committee rejected this on the grounds that it put patients at risk of heart attacks. Dr D was aware of the risk, and thought that he had suggested adequate safeguards in the research protocol. But what annoyed him was the suggestion that a GP would not have the scientific skills to carry out an accurate measurement of CO_2 levels. 'Surely I have been adequately trained in science as a doctor!'

6.2   Criticism of the preclinical curriculum

Having been selected by the methods and criteria already described, the medical student embarks on the preclinical part of the medical curriculum: typically two (sometimes three) years of study focused around the traditional 'basic medical sciences' of anatomy, physiology, and biochemistry: together with a course in the social sciences related to medicine (various combinations of subjects such as psychology, sociology, social policy, public health, and philosophy). There may or may not be some early clinical experience; but this is not the primary focus of the course.

In considering the preclinical curriculum, the need for change seems obvious to many commentators: indeed there have been calls for reform ever since the preclinical part of medical training reached its present structure during the late nineteenth century (see Chapter 2).

Criticism is typically focused upon content, volume, and form. The present curricular content is considered to be largely irrelevant to the vocational needs of doctors; there is simply too much of it; and it is taught in a manner which is both boring and conceptually unchallenging. Criticisms of the irrelevance of the early years have been made for generations (to little effect) but the conceptually unchallenging nature of the course has been the crucial complaint in recent years. Earlier generations of medical students were selected from the general run of 'grammar school' boys primarily by their ability to pay and by their vocation. But the greatly increased popularity of medicine among school-leavers has resulted in a striking rise in the academic abilities of medical students, who frequently regard themselves as the intellectual élite among university students (vet schools, with the highest entrance requirement of all, being both smaller and less common than medical schools).

Students are therefore startled and disappointed when they discover that the major difficulties of early medicine are in remembering a large volume of information — all the elements of which are, however, easy to understand on a fact-by-fact basis: a task somewhat akin to the memorizing of nonsense-words that psychologists use as a pure test of memory because it does not allow the higher mental functions of logic and reasoning to 'interfere' with the memory process.

In an uncontroversial sense, much of the preclinical curriculum is obviously valuable, and even essential — doctors must know their way around the visible parts of the human body, the names of the clinically important bits and pieces, and roughly what they do. This kind of familiarity with biology is an essential background, a true foundation on which the science is built, and upon which the practice of medicine constantly draws. But there is an increasing body of objective evidence to confirm the strong (if not universal) impression that the great bulk of what is taught (and particularly, what is *examined*) is neither retained, nor useful. There seems to be a gradual process of forgetting 'rote-learned' preclinical material which is proportional to the length of time which has elapsed since it was studied. This implies that the material is not being used, not being reinforced; and also that the knowledge is not necessary for clinical practice of even the highest standard. This much is also relatively uncontroversial.

None the less, it is usually claimed by supporters of the status quo that having gone through the process of learning a mass of detailed medical science the student retains it in a latent form, and this both facilitates future learning and, even more importantly, provides a conceptual framework, a way of thinking and reasoning, which is then applicable to later clinical work. However, a series of papers from Patel and co-workers have strongly suggested, using a number of sophisticated investigative strategies, that the 'scientific' and 'clinical' ways of thinking do not intersect significantly, and that they may be considered to be completely distinct knowledge structures or knowledge-bases. In other words clinicians do not actually use scientific concepts in diagnosis and treatment; and, if they do, then those concepts often prove to be misleading, and result in inappropriate action. The results of these studies 'challenge the generally accepted assumption that clinical medicine and basic science form an integrated knowledge domain'. Instead the preclinical science and clinical practice form separate domains, autonomous and connected only at discrete points. Such findings explain why preclinical students seem to 'know nothing' when they get on to the wards: and why the theories of medicine — presented in terms of systematic and 'scientific' schemes — are so much less useful than simple rules of thumb when it comes to managing clinical problems. So the justification of the present preclinical curriculum in terms of providing a foundation for vocational training has begun to look unconvincing — it seems clear that most of what is taught is not of value in clinical medicine.

6.3   Scientific method

But vocational training is not everything. As we have already argued, there should be broader perspectives in an undergraduate curriculum — those elements which can be called 'education' in contrast to 'training'. These, it is suggested, encompass features related to a broad cognitive perspective integral to the subject, so that it is of wide-ranging interest and applicability, can act to shape and transform an individual's outlook in a positive sense. Accordingly, the preclinical curriculum is often justified as being a scientific education for medical students.

If we accept that a good education in the methods of science is the best justification for a distinct preclinical period of study, we must ask to what extent this is being achieved. Is preclinical science good science? Is it taught in an appropriate fashion to produce an educated student? The first thing we notice is that science is taught differently in medical schools from the way it is taught in science faculties. In a nutshell, in medicine the students are taught *about* science, instead of *how to do* science; taught scientific knowledge, instead of the methods and skills of science. This is partly a result of the extremely broad coverage of subjects, and partly the result of the teaching methods used (textbooks, lectures, and demonstrations/practicals). Honours science graduates have a variable 'foundation' in such bread-and-butter knowledge; but their real 'education' in science comes from the kind of grappling with the primary stuff of science (papers, seminars, experiments) which they get through project work in the later years of the degree. It is from this latter kind of study that skills such as critical evaluation, hypothesis formation, judgement, and the presentation of conclusions are allowed the chance to develop. But in medicine, just at the point when a sixth-former has learned enough to proceed to the educative aspects of physics, chemistry, and biology, he or she is forced to drop them and start on the elements of a new series of subjects, viz. anatomy, physiology, and biochemistry.

6.4　Pragmatic justifications

The striking way in which the preclinical curriculum is widely recognized to be broadly deficient in both clinical relevance and educational atmosphere leads on to a consideration of just what its positive qualities might be. After all, if there was nothing to be said in its favour the curriculum would surely have been reformed before now. There are two powerful justifications for traditional modes of preclinical training: one explicit and the other implicit.

The justification which is most commonly explicitly advanced is that it gives an opportunity to 'weed out' the weaker and less motivated students at an early stage. But perhaps the implicit function is more important. It is easy to forget just what a terrifying thing it is to be a doctor. The responsibility for preserving life and health may be one which weighs heavily on a sensitive individual; and so the medical profession has developed a method of sharing this weight of responsibility. The method involves an intense and powerful process of professionalization. The first way in which the groundwork is prepared has traditionally been by providing an atmosphere in which a strong sense of corporate identity is encouraged. The medical class is physically together for many hours; they share a heavy workload and the ordeals of examination; and they may be geographically secluded from other groups of students. Some of their experiences (for example dissection classes) may be unusually stressful. So that the experience at medical school bears some resemblance to army basic training, and has some of the same goals: to induce toughness, to reduce sensitivity (otherwise known as 'squeamishness'), and to encourage the efficient use of time, respect for the profession, and an acceptance of hierarchy. It is in this sense that the traditional preclinical curriculum may be regarded as an apt vocational preparation for the current realities of working in most medical specialties.

On the other hand, whatever its pragmatic justifications, such an approach can hardly be defined as educational in the sense in which universities are supposed to operate. Such reasoning leads logically to an attempt to replicate, or even surpass, the gruelling fatigue of days and nights 'on call' at the earliest opportunity! Instead, it might be more reasonable to ensure that the early years of the preclinical training are distinct from clinical practice, and that we encourage individuality rather than identification with the professional group, critical thought rather than acceptance of hierarchical authority, and the rationality of science rather than the empiricism of medicine.

6.5   Devising a core curriculum

We then begin to see the possibility of a new pattern. If, on the one hand, the great mass of current preclinical teaching is without significant vocational training value other than in a negative sense; and, on the other hand, we lack space in the timetable to develop a truly educative scheme for scientific method, we have a case for arguing that the preclinical curriculum should therefore be reorganized in a rational manner to make it both more relevant and more interesting, and better adapted to the needs of training and of education alike.

The aim is to provide the vital 'basic medical science' knowledge required for clinical practice while simultaneously pursuing broader educational goals, mainly (although we hope not exclusively) through the promotion of a good scientific training. Limiting factors are related to logistical constraints. For example, it now seems to be clear that a fully 'vertically integrated' curriculum without the distinct preclinical–clinical division, and with basic science teaching largely done by active clinicians — however desirable — is not a realistic possibility for the already established medical schools, where there is neither the will nor the cash to do it. Furthermore, any proposals which require a higher level of recurrent funding, or have major implications for manpower allocation, are unlikely to get off the ground in the present or any foreseeable financial climate. This means that, for example, a universal lengthening of the degree to include an extra year with an intercalated B. Sc. is not a viable proposition (and anyway, leaves the problems of the existing curriculum untouched). We must do what we can to improve things using the time and people available — working with the existing two-year preclinical and three-year clinical degree, and with a mixture of scientists in the former and clinicians in the latter division.

The most difficult task is to devise a rational *core curriculum* for the preclinical years. We may be convinced that a much smaller segment of the two years will suffice to teach the medical students what they need to know; but the composition of this core is far from straightforward. Before we can devise a rational curriculum, we must devise 'objective' methods to decide what should go into it.

A present there is no 'method' — rather the implicit technique is to gather a few 'wise men' (professors and other heads of department) into a room and let them sort it out. The curriculum is then the accidental result of multiple collisions between various dominant personalities defending departmental vested interests, modified by Machiavellian 'horse-trading' and held in check only by the inertia of tradition. Having broadly divided the timetable into segments on the basis of departments or courses, the details of what is actually taught are determined on the basis of the subject requirements in the first place, with any vocational links put in later as added spice. For example, the subject of anatomy describes and interrelates what is seen in the dissection room (aiming for completeness, with emphasis placed on the structurally important), and this may then be followed by a few anecdotes about the clinical importance of a few of the things previously discussed (which are not necessarily the parts of anatomical importance). In other words anatomy is primary, clinical relevance is secondary, and the curriculum is decided by anatomists. This is precisely the wrong way round for a vocational course. A truly vocational training must start with *the job*, and move back to the basics needed to understand what happens in good practice. In other words, to return to our example, core course anatomy should be taught in a way and to a level which promotes an understanding of what is experienced in clinical practice. This means that vocational curriculum planning should in this sense be a 'top-down' process. It should flow, not from the traditional methods, skills, and boundaries of the preclinical sciences, but from the requirements of practice — which can surely best be established by consultation with excellent and active clinicians.

Harden (1986) has outlined possible rational techniques which would appear to offer an improvement on the 'wise men' method, such as defining a population of 'ideal' clinicians (or 'star performers') in the key specialties from which the curriculum is to be derived, and then questioning them in detail about their practice and/or studying them at work ('task analysis').

This is less straightforward than it might seem. To begin with, there will inevitably be disagreement as to the composition of the key specialties — although surveys of recent medical graduates show considerable agreement as to which clinical specialties are the most important (viz. medicine, surgery, paediatrics, obstetrics and gynaecology, emergency medicine, and general practice). Then again, it is unlikely that clinicians could, without considerable guidance and reflection, spontaneously volunteer a valid account of the range and content of basic medical science knowledge which underpins their practice. Such knowledge may be so obvious to them that it is not reported (for example, the names of the big bones) or else so specific to the specialty of particular consultants that they omit to mention the item (for example, neurosurgeons' detailed knowledge of cerebral circulation). However, while acknowledging the difficulties, it would seem that broadly speaking this is the manner in which we should proceed. Clearly, one starting-point would be to devise semi-structured questionnaires and interview schedules which would be completed by selected teams of key specialty clinicians and which would give a baseline of knowledge from which a core curriculum could be constructed.

A further technique which could be applied to the same population would be critical incident technique. This was originally devised for use in training armed forces personnel, but has since been adapted for use in a number of medical situations. In essence, the technique starts by isolating 'critical incidents', which are those discrete parts of a job where intervention is clearly effective and important — for example, diagnoses which must not be missed, efficacious treatments, or key features of management plans. These incidents are then subjected to analysis in terms of the skills and knowledge required to make those effective interventions, and these skills and knowledge can then be made the focus of training procedures.

The critical incident technique clearly has the advantage of teaching what is necessary for specific tasks of proven value, and may therefore have a role in medicine where certain situations are common and the appropriate action is well understood. Obviously, the technique is labour-intensive; and equally obviously it does not begin to encompass the whole of what being a good doctor is about. However, the 'art of medicine' is not the subject of any curriculum, but is learned by working closely and over a sustained period (like an apprentice) with a respected senior upon whom students can model themselves. Therefore, critical incident theory would form a legitimate part — but only a part — of the range of techniques for rational curriculum construction.

6.6 Teaching and examining

Having determined what should be taught to ensure a competent clinician ripe for postgraduate specialization there is clearly room for debate and divergence about how this knowledge is taught, in what order, and under what subject headings. This could vary between different medical schools, taking account of their traditions and internal organization.

There are also implications for examinations. If we have constructed a truly valid core curriculum, then it is reasonable to expect that students should attain mastery of the entire corpus of that material. Instead of, as at present, teaching more than students can take in, and then expecting them to recall about half of it (a fifty per cent pass mark), we would teach what they actually needed to know, and then expect them to remember virtually all of it (reaching a higher than ninety per cent pass mark). This knowledge should be easy to retain, because it is derived primarily from the basic science that clinicians use, and thus is constantly being reinforced by practice.

The need for research before defining a core curriculum leads on to the further consideration that this process would clearly be a major task; initially, at least, beyond the resources of any individual medical school. Equally it is a task which would fit well into medical research as it is practised at present, breaking up into publishable chunks. Research could be undertaken piecemeal, analysing expert skills on a subject-by-subject basis, and be published in the appropriate specialist journals. For example, analysis of the skill of a general surgeon and the basic science background to them could be undertaken by a surgical trainee as an MD project. This approach may have advantages in commanding respect from clinicians.

The most rational approach might be to do the job nationally, and to make the results generally available. Once the parameters of a core curriculum had been defined by a process of analysis such as that outlined above, then it would only be necessary to build in a system for updating and revising. This would involve much less work, and could consist of a forum for suggestions and criticisms, which would alert the national regulatory body to changes in clinical practice which had implications for basic science teaching. It would seem logical that such a regulatory body should come under the umbrella of the General Medical Council.

It is obvious that a national core curriculum could provide a mechanism for enforcing a national standard between medical schools — if such a standard is seen as lacking under the present system of loosely-interlocking external examiners. There could be improvements in efficiency and objectivity if the examination of this part of the curriculum were set and marked nationally. It should be a simple matter to condense the required knowledge into a single recommended textbook, which could be produced cheaply, and kept constantly under revision.

6.7 Project work

But we must not lose sight of the major reason for proposing such a national core curriculum, which is not efficiency or the regulation of standards, but the improvement of medical education. The core curriculum would substitute a short but highly relevant curriculum for the present long and largely irrelevant curriculum. And the reason for this is to allow space for a proper scientific education. Freed from the requirement of complete coverage, science teaching in medicine could rapidly move to a depth where students are working from primary materials (papers in journals and their own experiments or those of their supervisors) rather than from lectures and textbooks. Freed from the great bulk of bread-and-butter teaching, the staff would have the time and energy to supervise them.

In essence this work would be project-based. There is something to be said for a variety of projects in completely different types of medical science (for example, anatomy, cell biology, and community health); and there is also a good case to be made for a single topic of study, which could be written up as a thesis and/or a paper. Subjects studied could range through any of the current preclinical disciplines, and could probably also include clinical subjects, or even subjects outside the science faculty altogether in approved cases (subjects drawn for example from the social sciences, the humanities, or the law). Such project work would give students just that element of apprenticeship, of 'contagion' with seniors who have the appropriate attitude, which will be so important during their clinical years, and which is currently so lacking during their preclinical studies. This apprenticeship is potentially a highly sophisticated learning process, appropriate for passing on both skills and patterns of thought.

Project work would be highly conceptually challenging when compared with the present requirement for memorization skills; and the students would be assessed and graded on the basis of their scientific performance. Any reasonably motivated student should sail through the core curriculum exam, which would not, therefore, be discriminatory — but rather a minimum standard of competence, analogous to the medical 'examination' to get into the army, which everyone 'passes' unless there is a very good reason for them not to.

This kind of preclinical curriculum would answer the common criticism of lack of depth in medical training, which amounts to a lack of medical 'education' — every student would end up as a 'mini-expert' in at least one aspect of his or her studies. Which particular aspect does not really matter, as an education in scientific method and self-directed study would be broadly applicable, and would remain useful for the rest of the doctor's career.

6.8   Dual purpose of preclinical science

We are proposing that the preclinical curriculum has a dual purpose, both strictly vocational and broadly educational, and that these purposes can best be attained by separating them. We also propose that the preclinical period has a distinctive goal of its own, which is focused on the task of educating students in the skills of science. Emphasis would shift from the theory to the practice of science. The reforms we suggest are a combination of devising a core curriculum of the relevant vocational knowledge (perhaps nationally regulated and examined) and using the bulk of the timetable thus liberated for project work in science. The result would be a reduction in the variability between medical schools with regard to basic, essential teaching; but an increase in diversity with regard to exposing the students to some of the varied scientific specialties at which different universities excel.

Although the core curriculum proposal requires research input initially, once established the system would not require any alteration in funding or manpower. Teaching methods are already well established, since they are those used for a good B.Sc. degree. Indeed, the system is likely to be more popular than the present one among academic staff, as it gives increased opportunity for 'high level' teaching, with the possible benefits of discussing and doing research alongside highly qualified and motivated medical students. Students are likely to benefit from closer interaction with scientists in specialties which they can choose for themselves; they may also develop a long-term scientific interest, and publish material of their own in their chosen fields.

6.9 Conclusions

1. We began the chapter with a frank statement of the widely felt dissatisfaction with the preclinical teaching of science.

2. Such dissatisfaction, as exemplified by Miss B. our medical student, and such scientific weakness, as exemplified in Dr D, our over-ambitious GP, are at least partly a product of the character of the existing preclinical science curriculum.

3. We then tried to develop a critique of the preclinical curriculum and to suggest positively how it should be amended to make it at once more scientific, more clinically relevant, and more educational.

Bibliography

Charlton, B. G. (1991). Practical reform of preclinical education: core curriculum and science projects. *Medical Teacher*, **13**, 21–8.

Harden, R. M. (1986). *Ten questions to ask when planning a course or curriculum*. Association for the Study of Medical Education, Dundee.

Lancet (Editorial) (1988). Critical questions, critical incidents, critical answers. *Lancet*, **i**, 1373–4.

Newman, C. (1957). *The evolution of medical education in the nineteenth century*. Oxford University Press, London.

Patel, V. L. Evans, D. A., and Groen, G. J. (1989). Reconciling basic science and clinical reasoning. *Teaching and Learning in Medicine*, **I**, 116–21.

Wright, V., Hopkins, R., and Burton, K. E. (1979). What shall we teach undergraduates? *British Medical Journal*, **279**, 805–7.

7 The preclinical curriculum: social sciences and humanities

7.1 Some cases

7.1.1

Dr M. is a paediatrician who is explaining to a class of final-year medical students the nature and treatment of osteomyelitis. The seven-year-old boy he has been treating has been feverish, but has coped well, and his mother has agreed that the two of them should appear in front of the class while Dr M. is teaching. In the course of his teaching Dr M. indicates that while he hopes to treat the problem medically he intends taking his young patient to a surgeon, and he says to the class 'You know what surgeons are like when they get a knife in their hands.' The class duly laugh. The small boy is upset, and when the mother later taxes the paediatrician with his tactless remarks she is told 'You've got to make a few jokes or students get bored.'

7.1.2

Dr R. has begun a 'rotation' to become a GP. This involves three months at a hospice. In preparation for this she has read several books on death and dying, and is aware that there are typical stages that patients go through when they learn that they have a terminal illness — denial, anger, and so on. The consultant explains that patient S. has been told that she has a terminal illness. At first the patient could not believe it, but now seems cheerfully resigned. Dr R. is convinced that patient S. is bottling up her anger, and tries to give her an opportunity to express this. She then comes to realize that patient S. is not at all angry, and is in fact cheerfully resigned.

7.2 Medicine and 'whole-person care'

It has been recognized for several decades that medicine is not just about illness and disease, but is also about caring for and sometime even curing human beings who have illnesses and diseases. As soon as the importance of 'whole-person care' is acknowledged then the curriculum must include some disciplines which are concerned with human beings as a whole and in their social environment. To cover this aspect of patient-care many medical courses have created some room in the curriculum for the social sciences. The case for this is easy to make, since the social sciences seem to be concerned with the wider aspects of human behaviour, and since such subjects can be entered under the heading of 'science'. For example, psychology or (to ensure its relevance) 'clinical psychology' is a familiar component of a medical curriculum, and more recently medical sociology has been included. It is much harder to make out a case for the 'humanities' (philosophy, literature, and history) although, as we have already pointed out (Chapter 2) they were the earliest components in the education of the 'gentleman' doctor. We shall spend most time in this chapter in arguing for a limited return of such subjects to the curriculum, or at least to the education of doctors. Such subjects are just as relevant to the educated doctor as the social sciences, and we stress their importance not just because they make for the cultivated doctor, but because they contribute very largely to that important approach to care to which all doctors pay lip-service — whole-person understanding.

The case for the humanities is in fact easy to state in general terms. There are three main aspects to a good doctor: knowledge, skills, and a certain humane and wise attitude to patients. Knowledge is developed all through the curriculum and also in specialized and continuing medical education. Skills are also developed all through, but especially from the clinical years on. Medical knowledge and skills, which are of course interdependent, are developed by means of the study and practice of the medical and the social sciences. But *attitudes* are left undeveloped and unquestioned.

It might be argued that the social sciences are concerned with individual and social attitudes. This is true; but they have three limitations for the purposes we currently have in mind. First, the social sciences, by their very nature as sciences, must be concerned with *typical* behavioural or attitudinal patterns, whereas whole-person care is concerned with *uniqueness*, with what it means for a given patient to have a health problem. Secondly, the social sciences, again by their nature as sciences, encourage *detachment* from their subjects, whereas whole-person care requires involvement. Thirdly, the social sciences are concerned with the attitudes of *others* — patients, deprived groups, the bereaved, etc. — rather than with the *doctor's own attitudes* to his

patients, which are essential to whole-person care. The humanities are particularly appropriate for remedying all three
deficiencies of the social sciences. Indeed, the 'medical humanities' are a recognized part of medical education in the USA and
elsewhere. In order to develop these points let us first look at
the kind of understanding provided by the sciences and the
social sciences.

7.3   Understanding: science and social science

Let us begin by considering what it is to understand an event in
a scientific manner. To understand an event is to be able to fit it
into a pattern or system of similar events. The natural sciences
are concerned with discovering the types of pattern or uniformity in terms of which natural events can be understood. Obviously, patterns or orders of many varieties can be traced in
nature, from the microscopic to the macroscopic. From another
point of view we could say that nature can be ordered in different ways according to the purposes of the scientist. Sometimes
these orders are at the level of classifications. For example, the
basis on which the medical scientist begins his investigations is
the series of classifications which we call biology. The development of science can be depicted as the process of tracing ever
finer patterns or orders in nature, and scientific understanding
is then a matter of fitting events or phenomena into these
patterns. It is of great interest in the philosophy of science how
far these patterns are discovered in nature and how far they are
imposed by the scientist on nature; but the idea of systematic
patterns (or theories) is common to both ways of looking at the
development of science.

A second feature of scientific understanding should be noted.
Sometimes the phenomena to be understood are of very great
complexity, and the scientist is unsure of the systematic
connections in the pattern. In this situation understanding can
be created by the development of a model, or a simplified
pattern, which ignores some of the complexities. Models in this
sense are theoretical templates.

A fuller account of scientific understanding would require a
discussion of the place of observation and experiment, hypotheses, and the many different sorts of patterns which are

characteristic of different sciences; but this crude account is sufficient for present purposes.

Turning now to the social sciences, we find that an account of the understanding of human action is presupposed which is similar to the scientific understanding of events and processes. The social sciences attempt to trace the patterns or systems which shape human wants and objectives. Some of these patterns are economic, some political, some legal, some religious or ideological, some psychological. Knowledge of these patterns is undoubtedly of great assistance in understanding human behaviour in general terms. Like the natural sciences, the social sciences also use hypotheses and models, such as 'rational economic man'.

In tracing the patterns into which human behaviour tends to fall, social scientists frequently use the term 'social role', as we have done. While there is no unambiguous use of the concept, far less a single definition of it, it is a useful tool of social science, in that it can act as a bridge concept to explain the influence of society on the conduct of the individual. Thus, individuals act in society as labourers, builders, musicians, farmers, teachers, doctors, probation officers, or fathers, where these terms indicate a social function. While individuals act in these roles, thus contributing to the maintenance of society, the roles in turn shape and influence the whole personalities of the persons who act in them. A knowledge of the social sciences is therefore essential for any adequate understanding of individual action, because the influence of society is present in every individual action.

Nevertheless, there are serious limitations to this approach as a way of attaining 'whole-person' understanding. First of all, an undue emphasis on one social science can distort our view of human behaviour. For example, it is accepted in social science that economic influences are exceedingly important in shaping human behaviour, whether that of individuals, groups, or nations. But 'rational economic man' is an abstraction, and does not correspond to any actual person. People do not often, if ever, act from purely economic motives — or at least it is a simplistic assumption that they always do; someone may well sacrifice an economic gain for reasons of social status, love, spitefulness, high moral principle, religious zeal, or revenge.

Of course, a doctrinaire social scientist might reply that all these apparently diverse motives can alike be classified as 'preferences' and measured economically; but this move encourages us to see uniformity in human motivation where there is in fact complexity. People certainly act in social roles, but not just in one; and the difficulty in applying social science to human behaviour is that of knowing the relevance of the different frames of reference of the different social sciences. Nothing brings the social sciences into greater disrepute than the pretensions of one social scientist — a Freudian psychologist, or a Marxist economist, say — to explain all human behaviour in terms of a few simplistic concepts. This can be said without at all decrying the great explanatory power of both Freudian psychology and Marxist economics. While a knowledge of the different patterns elaborated in the social sciences is a help in understanding human behaviour, these patterns are abstractions from the complex reality of individual human conduct, and since the doctor, nurse, dentist, and social worker are concerned with this individual, or this family group, or this neighbourhood, there are limits to the explanatory power of social science, and dangers of distortion in the uncritical use of scientific frames of reference.

There is also a second sort of limitation to the explanatory power of the social sciences as they apply to human behaviour. To bring this out let us consider the connection between being a person and having a role. It might first be suggested that the relationship is one of identity, in the sense that acting as a person just is acting as an X, or Y, or Z, where these last name a social role. If this thesis were valid, then, subject to the difficulties already mentioned of knowing which explanatory frameworks to apply, it would be possible to have a complete explanation of human behaviour in terms of one or more of the social sciences. For there can be detailed objective descriptions of the roles which people play.

This account, however, omits to mention one essential aspect of every action — the choice requirement. People can choose to accept or reject their roles; they are not fixed by them. Moreover, while playing the role of doctor, social worker, teacher, nurse, father, trade unionist, etc., a person can become detached from his roles, and can laugh at himself in them. This suggests that there is an important personal dimension to action which is not caught by the concept of a social role. In other words, to understand an action it is important to know how the person him/herself sees the action, and more generally what his/her attitude is to the role. And understanding of this kind does not come from applying any social science.

Thirdly and most fundamentally of all, the understanding which comes from depicting human behaviour in terms of patterns can never, even in principle, provide us with 'whole-person' understanding. It is the wrong sort of understanding. To understand in terms of patterns is to find similarities, and this is a valid perspective. But the 'whole-person' perspective is concerned with uniqueness. For example, to understand Mrs Green from a 'whole-person' perspective is to be concerned not with her *likeness* to other behaviour patterns but with her *this-ness*. Knowledge of patient behaviour (the role of the patient) may be a help in understanding Mrs Green (although, as we shall see, it may also be a hindrance); but it does not give us any understanding of what it is for Mrs Green to exhibit this behaviour.

7.4 Understanding: history and the arts

The social sciences are not the only means of providing understanding of human action: historians and biographers can also do so. Historians and biographers give us understanding of human actions by telling the story, as factually accurate as possible, which enables us to understand how particular persons came to act as they did. Of course, the simple reporting of a set of actions does not by itself provide understanding; understanding occurs when we perceive the motivational links between actions and events in the lives of the individuals we are studying.

It is important to note the difference between this sort of historical and biographical understanding and that provided by the social sciences. The social sciences are concerned with similarities and with repeatable patterns. In contrast, historical and biographical understanding is created by the exploration of the policies, values and motivation of one person through a period of time. In their concern with the sequences of actions of particular people the historian and biographer are therefore concerned with what is unique and unrepeatable.

Does it follow from the previous section that whole-person understanding is achieved through biography or history (or the medical and nursing version of this, which is the case history or the patient's story)? Certainly, biography and history are concerned with unique individuals, and such concerns enable us to take a vital step towards whole-person understanding. But it might be possible to have this sort of understanding of a person without its counting as whole-person understanding. Take the example of a patient who is HIV-positive. A doctor might have scientific understanding of this patient in terms of his knowledge of the relevant disease patterns. He might further be assisted in his understanding by his knowledge of the typical patterns of behaviour displayed by drug addicts. In addition, and more relevantly for present purposes, he might acquire understanding from his knowledge of the case history of this particular patient. For example, he might have learned that the patient's rejection at home and at school led him to keep company with drug addicts, and have inferred that the sharing of needles was for this patient the only sort of sharing he had ever experienced. But a doctor or nurse who came in this way to understand the patient through science, social science, and case history might nevertheless condemn, be judgemental, and remain on the outside of the patient's story. This would be a sign that whole-person understanding is lacking; such doctors or nurses would not be 'understanding' people. What is lacking?

The answer is that what is lacking is the understanding of the *meaning* of this biography for the patient. And it is in the understanding of meaning for a person that we find the final ingredient in whole-person understanding. Involved in this sort of understanding are the abilities to *interpret* a set of actions or a personal story from the point of view of the person telling it, and also the ability to *feel* with the person whose story it is. Sometimes the term 'empathy' is used in this context; but the danger of such a word is that it suggests something technical, that only the caring professions know how to do. The truth is rather that it is an ability which all normal people have, and indeed it is perhaps less conspicuous in the caring professions than in humbler mortals, for the reason that the caring profession are inclined to regard its ordinary manifestations as unscientific and unprofessional, and so pretend it is something technical by calling it 'empathy'. Be that as it may, our claim is that the final component of whole-person understanding has both a cognitive element — an ability to interpret the meaning of action from the perspective of another person — and an emotional element — an ability to feel with that person. It involves imaginative and intuitive insight into the meaning of another person's experience, coupled with a compassion for the person whose experience it is.

In pulling together the threads of this account of the meaning of the expression 'whole-person understanding' we must guard against some misinterpretations. First, it is true that the final component in whole-person understanding — the compassionate insight into meaning — is the most important — so much so that someone who displays such imaginative insight and fellow-feeling is often called an 'understanding person'. Nevertheless, our thesis does not require that the term 'whole-person understanding' be arrogated to the last component on its own. On the contrary, our thesis is that whole-person understanding is the outcome of the totality of the four different modes of understanding: the scientific, the social, the case history, and the imaginatively felt insight into meaning. The interpretation of the patient's story, to be appropriate, must be based on a correct diagnosis and an accurate case history.

In the second place, it is important to remember that people are part of larger social units. The expression 'whole-person understanding' has an individualistic sound to it. But it is usually impossible to understand the meaning of other people's experience without knowing something of their social context.

Thirdly, more than one interpretation of the meaning of someone's experience may be possible. In telling their story, via their case history or otherwise, patients may be seeking to make sense of their experience or to give some meaning to their suffering. They may ask 'Why me?', and try to answer the question. It is in this context that a carer can sometimes help, by suggesting new ways of looking at the event. There can be more than one way of giving meaning to someone's life.

Fourthly, the process of seeking meaning in another person's story is one which obviously involves one's own values. It is true in social science that one's own values may affect one's findings; and likewise in history or biography the personality of the writer enters into his description of what he sees. It is even more the case that the personality of the carer is involved in the search for meaning in the story of another person.

Finally, people are not fixed by their stories. A life story is not like a Greek drama, proceeding with a dramatic necessity to an inevitable conclusion. We can 'fix' someone with their story when in fact they have moved on to another chapter which does not cohere with the previous one, and indeed which alters the meaning of the previous one. There is nothing immutable about meaning, and therefore whole-person understanding is not an achievement, but an unending process.

7.5   Achieving and teaching 'whole-person understanding'

The argument has been that 'whole-person understanding' is an amalgam of the understanding which comes from the sciences, the social sciences, a detailed case history, and compassionate insight into the meaning of the case history for a particular patient in his/her social context. How can such understanding be achieved and taught? In answering this question we shall at the same time be expanding the analysis of the concept of this sort of understanding.

We have already discussed in Chapter 6 the idea of education through the biological sciences. These are familiar aspects of medical and nursing education. The relevant difficulty is with the idea of understanding the meaning of people's actions from their own perspective and feeling with them. How can that be achieved and taught?

One answer might be that people already have (or do not have) the ability in question, and that therefore it cannot either be acquired or taught. In replying to this objection we need not deny that some people are much better by nature than others at achieving imaginative insights into the minds and feelings of others. All that is necessary is to insist that we all do have the ability to some degree, and that it can be developed and its importance can be emphasized. How?

The disciplines which develop and extend this catalytic component of whole-person understanding are above all history and literature in all its aspects. Indeed, they may be more effective in preparing doctors and nurses for responding to patients than the social sciences, which encourage labelling and stereotyping. The humanities, rather than the social sciences, are concerned with the *particularity* of situations and with their *meaning*, and that concern is the way to whole-person understanding. In this section we shall concentrate on the contribution of literature.

Novels, plays, poems, films, or paintings can make a large impact on a student or doctor, and help to develop intuitive understanding. Heaven forbid that the arts should be studied only because they are useful; but a study of the arts is educative because it is able to provide insight into the particularity of situations. Whereas science, including social science, proceeds by induction from specific instances to generalized (often idealized) patterns, the arts concentrate on the concrete details of specific situations and through the exploration of these details they can bring out the underlying meaning in human predicaments. Study of this sort is more relevant to the concerns of a doctor, nurse, or social worker than is the study of the more abstract disciplines of sociology, psychology, or philosophy.

For example, there is a surprising amount of poetry and other literature dealing with mental handicap. This is perhaps the case because the creative imagination responds to the ambiguous nature of the mentally handicapped person. Thus, the 'fool' who has profound insights because of his simplicity, who remains blameless in a corrupt world, who is both comic and tragic, who inspires both possessive love and repugnance, or who is a challenge to respectable values, is an obvious source of fascination to creative writers. A study of Wordsworth's 'The Idiot Boy' illustrates theoretical points about mental handicap with the immediate impact of poetry. Again, Jon Silkin's poem 'Death of a Son' (who died in a mental hospital, aged one) expresses more clearly than any treatise the attitudes of a parent towards the life and death of a mentally handicapped child.

In more detail, the study of the arts — poetry, the novel, drama, painting — can he helpful in three different ways to those dealing with illness. To begin with, it can both extend and also give cognitive shaping to the sympathetic imagination. The point here is that in dealing with illness, the social sciences, if they are to be sciences or respectable academic disciplines, must stand back from the phenomena and present their accounts in the detached prose style of science. On the other hand, the arts involve us directly, and makes us vividly and emotionally aware of what it is like to be in the situation the social scientist discusses. The arts develop and extend our sympathies, and make us feel something of what it is like to be a relative or a helper of someone who is ill. They may even provide some feeling of what it means to *be* handicapped or ill. The arts therefore develop sympathy of the passive or empathetic kind. Now, passive sympathy easily generates motivation to act, and active sympathy, however well-meaning, can be blind, clumsy, or humiliating unless it is informed by a sensitive understanding of particular situations or relationships. And the arts also have this other aspect, namely, that they can sensitize sympathy or give a cognitive shaping. In other words, imaginative literature or the arts generally can develop in a doctor or nurse a perception of real need.

Secondly, the arts can be a help in coming to terms with the emotions and conflicts which are released in anyone caring for those who are ill. The same is true of those dealing with problems of bereavement. Questions of the meaning of life, of the tragedy and tears built into human relationships, inevitably arise in such situations, and require some sort of answer if the life of professional care is to seem worth while. The arts can deal with these issues with an immediacy lacking in the abstractions of philosophy or social sciences.

Thirdly, the arts generate moral questions. It is a matter for theorists to discuss whether the arts ought to set out to be didactic, but it is in fact the case that good art does often give rise to moral questions. For example, in dramatizing a particular episode, literature can raise questions about the attitude of society to health problems, or it can challenge our own self-perceptions on these matters. Many medical courses nowadays contain teaching on medical ethics. This may be desirable, but unless the teaching is sensitively carried out it can simply become another set of technical terms or abstract principles which come between carers and their patients. The study of dramatic 'ethical dilemmas' may tax our intellects and provide TV discussion programmes, but the arts can force us to look beyond the false finalities of a textbook on ethics and challenge us to refashion our attitudes. It is not that the arts present us with some unrealistic idea, but rather that they explore for us the many facets of our ambiguous attitudes towards illness. When this happens, we find ourselves reconsidering the quality of our care and the nature of our social attitudes.

7.6   Is 'whole-person understanding' desirable?

It might be objected that what we are calling whole-person understanding is undesirable. The charge can take two forms. First, it might be objected that it is misguided to stress the importance for doctors and nurses of imaginative insight into the meaning of events and actions, because to do so is to emphasize what is unscientific, and medicine must be scientific.

In reply it must be pointed out that the sort of insight we are describing is *non-scientific*, (and therefore not *unscientific*). It is non-scientific because, as we have said already, scientific explanation and understanding is concerned with patterns; it is repeatable. On the other hand, the kind of understanding we are currently discussing is not repeatable, but is unique to each situation. But it does not follow from the point that imaginative insight is non-scientific either that it cannot be based on the evidence or that there is no way of testing it. The evidence will be a person's own accounts of how he sees his situation or his problems (it will be remembered that accurate diagnosis and case history are essential to whole-person understanding) and testing one's understanding of his/her reactions to further questions. A knowledge of social science might be a help here; but it is just as likely to be an impediment, because it will encourage the doctor to see unique individuals and their problems in terms of general categories and labels.

The term 'folk psychology' is sometimes invoked to disparage the kind of insights and understanding which come from the arts. The assumption seems to be that imaginative writers or artists are attempting to do crudely and unsystematically what modern psychologists do in a sophisticated and rigorous manner. This assumption need only be stated for its absurdity to be seen. Imaginative writers are not attempting to write systematic treatises on human behaviour, although this does not mean that what they write is not, in another sense, psychology. It is the term 'folk' that is objectionable in the expression, with its suggestion of unlearned naïvety. But the arts abound in refined, accurate, and sensitive identification and analysis of human beings and their relationships, and need not be at all simple-minded.

Can we learn from the arts? This innocent-seeming question conceals a dangerous dilemma. If we cannot learn from the arts then they must be seen as an amusing diversion or relaxation. This is indeed how many people, including many doctors, do see literature. The price for making this move, which many doctors would not regard as a high one, is that the arts cannot form part of a doctor's serious education. If, however, we take the other alternative and say that we can learn from the arts, then the argument becomes that the arts must therefore express repeatable elements in human experience. It can then be asserted that if the arts are concerned with repeatable elements they are doing unsystematically what the social sciences are trying to do scientifically, and we are back with the 'folk psychology' argument.

The answer to this is to insist that we can indeed learn from the arts, but deny that they teach us by generalizing from experience. The important question is not 'Can we learn from the arts?' but 'How do we learn from the arts?' The answer to the question thus reformulated is that we learn from the arts by imaginative identification with the situations or characters depicted, and by having our imaginations stretched through being made to enter into unfamiliar situations or to see points of view other than our own. Learning of this kind is generative of a deep understanding which is essential to humane doctoring.

The second form of the objection that whole-person understanding, as described in this chapter, is undesirable is based on a common assumption about the doctor–patient relationship — an assumption which we have ourselves made. The assumption is that by its very nature the doctor–patient relationship is a role-relationship, and not a personal one. It is considered a role-relationship for at least one good reason — that it is essential that doctors and nurses should be *detached* from patients and not personally involved with them, and to see the relationship as a role-relationship assists in the depersonalizing of it.

In reply one need not deny that the doctor–patient relationship is a role-relationship. But it is also a personal one; persons act in roles. This point becomes convincing if we reflect that a husband–wife relationship is a role relationship; clearly it can be and ought also to be a personal relationship involving whole-person understanding.

As for the implication that whole-person understanding may prevent 'distance' where that is necessary, we can simply deny that it does prevent distance. One important feature of whole-person understanding is that those who have it know when to be close and when to be detached. To return to the example of the husband and wife, it is obvious that whole-person understanding in that situation might involve the realization that detachment at the breakfast table is a good thing! In a similar way, the good doctor with a whole-person understanding of his patient will know when to be detached and when not. The insights of the arts develop this sort of sensitivity.

We have tried to provide an interpretation of the expression 'whole-person understanding' as it is used in a medical context. It should be noted that what we have proposed is not any dramatic changes in medical education, but rather a return to the ideals of a humane education. Most doctors pay lip-service to the view that medicine is an art as well as a science. Ignoring in this context the objection that most medical courses are not particularly scientific in the proper sense, this chapter has made a plea for the importance of the humanities in medicine and nursing. If whole-person understanding is an important concept in health care the humanities are important in medical education.

7.7 Ethics and communication skills

We have mentioned the importance for doctors of developing effective communication skills; but the decision of how and what to communicate is a moral matter. Certainly, there is much to be learned from the social science about the 'how', or the skill of communication. But communication skills ungoverned by moral attitudes become crude manipulation. What is needed in communication skills is not just technique, but a humane practice. Patients or clients can sense the difference between tact, charm, or sympathy which are simply 'turned on' as a matter of technique, and those which spring from a genuinely caring attitude.

Turning now to the question of what to communicate, we wish to emphasize that it is the individual doctor's *interpretation* of the available information which determines what is said to the patient. In making this point we are challenging the assumption that factual information in some scientifically compelling form is the only determinant of what to communicate. In most common medical or nursing problems the information available is not always 'firm', and judgement in choosing the appropriate course of action is almost always required. Hence the importance of the moral dimension in clinical decision-making as to what to communicate.

At this point two comments might be made about the consideration that there is a moral dimension in all clinical decisions. Both concede the importance of moral considerations in professional judgement. First, it could be said that the moral dimension is taken care of by requiring the student to learn the relevant code of ethics of the profession; and second, that the moral dimension is taken care of, not by learning, but by intuition, or, as some would have it, it is just a matter of 'common sense'. The second point might also be put by saying that since moral decisions are based on personal factors no guidelines could be drawn up to assist all health care professionals. Further, this attitude also implies that morality cannot be learned.

In replying to the first point we do not deny the importance of codes of ethics to a profession; but these are necessarily limited in scope, consisting only of broad principles which on occasion may even conflict with one another. Moreover, no set of principles can itself tell us how and when its constituent principles are to be applied in everyday life. Further, codes of ethics deal only with the profession's values — not with the patient's values, or the changing values of the wider society in which health care is practised.

In replying to the second point we can again agree with the importance of developing intuitive judgements in morality, as indeed in professional matters generally. The intuitions of an experienced practitioner in his or her field of work are likely to be better than those of an inexperienced person. But such intuitions, whether based on experience or not, may later need to be justified by appropriate observations and debate.

Consider a typical ward-round discussion of whether or not a 76-year-old man should be allowed home after a two-month admission because of a cerebrovascular accident which gave him temporary loss of function of the right arm and leg. After considerable rehabilitation it is now time to consider whether or not he should go home. Factual information will be available from tests and from the occupational therapist, the physiotherapist, and the social worker. Nursing and medical background will also be available. It is at this stage that the personal intuition of all will be brought into play.

In discussing the importance of 'intuitions' or 'hunches' in clinical decisions it is important to remember that just as our factual knowledge and skills require to be constantly upgraded, so the germs of social feeling which we may be born with require to be developed by use and extended by reason, and even our mature moral judgements require to be justified to others by argument; 'common sense' is not enough.

As we have stressed, literature can be of great help here. It is also important to bear in mind that literature, or the arts more generally, are concerned with the *particularity* of situations, with their *uniqueness*. But situations also have features in common, and can thus be governed by general principles or concepts. It is in the identification and analysis of the relevant moral principles and concepts that another of the humanities — philosophy — has a part to play in medical education. Let us now look at what medical ethics can contribute to the making of a doctor.

7.8   Medical ethics

There is a substantial literature on the general principles of medical ethics, as well as discussion of detailed problems within medical ethics. It is more appropriate in this context to consider how medical ethics may be taught and learned. We are none of us beginners in this. From infancy people learn and are taught morality by parents, schoolteachers, friends, colleagues, or television programmes. In that sense, then, learning about morality as a medical or nursing student is not like learning about biochemistry, where no previous knowledge can be presupposed. Moreover, our values change as we grow older; they are not fixed. But how can values be taught?

As a start in answering this question it is instructive to consider the traditional way of doing it, and to consider its defects. The traditional method — although 'method' is perhaps the wrong term, since it was never fully explicit — involved two stages. In the first stage, which usually took place early in the student's college or university years, some important and senior person would arrive and give a lecture or two on the relevant 'Code of Ethics', and then disappear and never be seen again. This had the effect of suggesting that ethics was something exalted and unconnected with one's everyday moral concerns.

The second stage took place during clinical teaching, and the idea was that the student acquired an 'ethical' grasp from observing the practice of an experienced professional. Just as the novice surgeon or the nursing student picks up knowledge and techniques from watching an experienced practitioner, so ethics was expected to be absorbed in much the same fashion. The stage, of course, presupposes that the senior's practice is exemplary, which it may not be, and that there is no room for other ways of looking at moral questions.

The basic assumption, common to both stages of the traditional method, is that explicit or implicit instruction must always be given exclusively by a senior member of the relevant profession — thus reinforcing the idea that 'ethics' is an occult matter, the mysteries of which are not for the layman or the inexperienced student. Criticism by outsiders of current practices is seen as 'doctor bashing' or 'nurse bashing', and the idea that the professional could sometimes learn from out-siders, or from juniors in the profession, is not thinkable.

This description is no doubt exaggerated, but has sufficient truth in it to warrant some suggestions for other ways of proceeding. We should like to suggest that the following factors are important for improving the teaching of morality in health care contexts, and therefore for improving health care. Attention must be given to:

(1)   the 'shape' of the teaching environment;

(2)   the content of what is taught;

(3)   how it is taught;

(4)   who teaches it; and

(5)   the example set in the hospital or any other care environment.

Whereas it is important that there should be lectures or other formal ways of teaching ethics in college or university, this teaching will come to nothing unless it is explicitly integrated with the practice experiences of the student, and is seen to be relevant. The teachers at each stage must know and refer to what has already been said, and above all the practitioners must take up relevant points and illustrate them. There should be co-ordination.

The content and method of teaching will depend on resources; but it is important to encourage critical discussion of a realistic sort. Thus a student might be asked to discuss a case, and to say what he would have done. Whereas much of the material for such discussions will involve case histories and moral philosophy, it is important to remember that novels, poems, plays, or films can make a large impact on a student, and develop the intuitive understanding we have stressed throughout the book.

Turning to the question of *who* should be involved in teaching medical ethics, we have found that it is helpful if the enterprise is a co-operative one with people outside the particular profession. For the professionals to do it all themselves gives a recipe for conservatism and whitewash; but if the classes are taken entirely by others then the students may not regard them with sufficient seriousness. Co-operations is essential, although not always easy to arrange. Moral philosophers, social scientists, and lawyers have an important place in teaching; so do patients and relatives, who can contribute a quite different slant on moral problems.

The final factor in moral education is the influence of seniors. Students will learn just as much or more from what is actually done in the real situation as from what is said. The teamwork between professionals of more than one discipline can be effective as an example in learning and teaching moral values.

In any teaching of medical ethics, especially where other disciplines such as philosophy or law are involved, it is important to keep in mind limited and realistic objectives. It is unrealistic to expect medical students to provide expositions of Utilitarianism, and not helpful to introduce technical terms, such as 'deontology', at an early stage. In our experience limited objectives, such as the following, are realistic:

1. *to make the students aware that decision-making in medicine is not value-free;*

2. *to assist the students in learning to deal with moral decision-making in a more rational way, by logic and argument, and to enable them to justify their own views and explore their own attitudes to moral problems, especially the relationship between personal and professional morality;* and

3. *to help the students to come to terms with conflict in ethical problems. This includes a consideration of the role of the doctor and the relationship with other members of the health team.*

These objectives can be pursued by the use of case studies, with the aim of articulating general principles.

There are three common problems raised by students in the use of case histories or practical examples in teaching. The first is the 'it depends' response. This view is that there are so many variables which are not given, and which would be required to make a decision, that it is not worth trying. The response would 'depend' on so many things that it is not possible even to discuss the issue.

The second problem is that the responses are so individual that discussion is irrelevant. This view makes the point that the subjective nature of the responses means that particular views on a topic are unlikely to change in a brief discussion.

The third problem is that before the question or case histories are discussed more professional knowledge or experience is required. The argument here is that only when you become a consultant, ward sister, etc., will you have sufficient background to tackle such questions. What is the point in trying, therefore?

These problems are important, and need to be considered further. Suppose students are asked to discuss the statement

'Patients over the age of seventy should not be resuscitated.' Clearly whether they agree or disagree with the statement *will* depend on many factors. The point of the exercise is to get them to think of the circumstances under which they would agree, or not. For example, they might agree to a resuscitation policy under the following conditions:

'Patients who have previously been well, with no other illnesses, with a good social environment and a supportive family';

and they could list conditions under which they would disagree with a resuscitation policy, such as:

'Multiple medical problems, no family support, etc.'

Equally, however, they could disagree with the approach that there *should* be guidelines for resuscitation, and maintain that it is morally wrong to have guidelines on this. They might broaden the discussion to raise the question as to who should make the decision.

The second concern about such statements is that responses are always personalized, and that within groups there could always be differences of opinion. But the point of discussion is not necessarily to achieve a consensus; it can also be to allow individual views to be heard, and to make participants aware that there may be more than one view on the subject. This is in order that:

(1) students can be clearer about their own views;

(2) they can develop understanding of the views of other, whether they be patients, relatives or staff; and

(3) they can compare their response with those of others with whom they disagree.

Point 3 is important. In professional life some doctors *will* disagree with others. Group discussion gives an opportunity to practise coping with disagreement.

The third concern often voiced in discussion is that it is impossible to answer many of the questions raised because students lack sufficient clinical experience. This view makes the assumption that greater experience, status, and knowledge can help to answer such questions. It also assumes that at a certain stage in one's career, the answers to ethical and moral questions become obvious. Now while there is no doubt that increasing clinical experience can change particular views, we need only consider the differences in views among senior members of professional groups to realize that experience alone will not ensure a consensus of opinion. Finally, students must remember that they may be faced with many of the situations described *before* they reach some elevated status, and they should therefore have a view on these matters now.

New knowledge, new techniques and new information are continually becoming available, and therefore professional experience will change with time. Most clinical decisions are based on information which is less than complete. Assumptions are made, and decisions are made on the basis of probabilities. There may be no certainty as to the outcome of a particular course of action. To delay taking moral decisions until all possible factual information is available is to misunderstand the nature of clinical decision-making.

It should be noted that we are not denying the importance of introducing students to the general principles and concepts of ethics, but stressing that they will seem remote and abstract unless they can be seen to arise out of specific cases to which students can relate. Statements and case histories should be seen as 'triggers' to discussion, and as stimuli for thought. They are essentially 'coat-pegs' on which to hand concepts and views.

7.9 Making space

It will be objected, even by those readers who have sympathy with our argument that the humanities can make an important contribution to medical education, that it is unrealistic to expect the curriculum to change sufficiently to make room for the humanities. And it is in any case true that many medical students will not respond well to humanities courses. Perhaps, then, any general culture which the doctor may succeed in acquiring after admission to medical school will have to be got outside the prescribed course of study. Unfortunately this may prove more than usually difficult in such a time-consuming curriculum, and one which places such a premium on passive learning and factual recall. And after qualification the problems are even worse. All of this is a serious indictment of medical education. On the one hand we have a public which, quite reasonably, expects an educated professional; while on the other hand the education provided not only omits virtually all potentially educational experience, but also largely *prevents* students acquiring such an education for themselves!

Fortunately there seems to be sufficient native talent in the medical intake that the situation is by no means lost, and there are remarkable numbers of cultivated individuals who, against the odds, manage to pursue activities broader than the strictly vocational; and these reflect credit on the medical profession as a whole. Some ideas for improving science education have already been described. It is probably unrealistic (and maybe unjustifiable) to expect much in the way of curricular expansion in non-scientific subjects. However, with such a highly selected and motivated population as present-day medical students, it seems entirely reasonable that even in 'the liberal arts' a great deal could be achieved by even a moderate degree of *encouragement* combined with an increased amount of time available for self-education. We believe that such efforts would be worth while precisely because, in so many ways, a medical education has so much to recommend it — producing a characteristic clarity of thought and unusually decisive capability for action. Such benefits cry out for completion and expansion into a broader and more humane world-view.

7.10   Conclusions

1. In this chapter we have made a case for the place of the social sciences, and more especially the humanities, in medical education. In particular we argue for the importance of the humanities in developing the appropriate attitudes which should provide the context in which the traditional medical skills are pursued. That context is one of 'whole-person understanding'.

2. 'Whole-person understanding' requires not only the scientific understanding of disease processes and of typical behaviour patterns, but also the understanding of the specifics of a given case history and the understanding of the meaning of that case history for the patient in question. It is the distinctive contribution of the humanities to medical

education to be able to develop the imaginative and perceptive insight into meaning.

3. More general philosophy or medical ethics can assist in the analysis and discussion of the value judgements which are all-pervasive in medical decision-making.

4. We can now see that in 7.1.1 Dr M lacks the awareness of what being a patient with a frightening ailment must mean to a young child. Dr R in 7.1.2 was over-impressed with sociological studies of patients who are given bad news. Medical sociology provides interesting information on typical patterns of reactions, but specific patients do not necessarily react in this way. Theory has come between her and the unique quality of this patient's reactions. Finally, it is well known that the continual care of patients can produce tension and psychological problems in doctors and nurses. This is especially true in some specialties, such as palliative medicine. Literature, art, and music can assist at least some doctors in coming to terms with such bottled-up reactions.

5. We recognize the difficulties of including courses in the humanities as part of the curriculum; but much can be done to create the space in which those who respond to the humanities can be given the opportunity to pursue such interests.

Bibliography

Brody, H. (1987). *Stories of sickness*. Yale University Press, New Haven–London.

Cassell, E. J. (1984). *The place of the humanities in medicine*. The Hastings Center, Hastings-on-Hudson, N.Y.

Charlton, B. G. (1991). Stories of sickness. *British Journal of General Practice*, **41**, 222–3.

Downie, R. S. (1991). Literature and medicine. *Journal of Medical Ethics*, **17**, 93–6.

Downie, R. S. and Calman, K. C. (1987). *Healthy respect*. Faber and Faber, London.

Gillon, R. (1987). *Philosophical medical ethics*. Wiley, Chichester.

8 Basic clinical education

8.1 A case

Mr J. has been a clinical medical student for the past year. During this time he has rotated through medicine (including cardiology, neurology, and diabetes), surgery (including orthopaedics, urology, and ophthalmology), psychiatry, paediatrics, and anaesthetics. While he has been well taught, and he has acquired an enormous amount of knowledge, he still feels unconfident about how to behave as a doctor. Also, he finds that not a single member of staff remembers his name.

8.2 The clinical undergraduate curriculum

In the preceding chapters we have expressed some serious doubts concerning the value of the preclinical section of medical training; by contrast it is widely accepted that the clinical curriculum — while far from perfect — is set up along more or less the right lines. As described in the introduction, we intend in this book to concentrate on those parts of the doctor's education which we regard as most deficient. We have now arrived at a part of medical education of established value; here, more than anywhere, is where the student learns to be a doctor. In this chapter, then, we shall be concerned with fine-tuning rather than radical rebuilding.

The clinical years are, like other aspects of education, variable between the different British medical schools; but they all conform to the description of a mixture of formal teaching with informal experiences (and, of course, private study) — of theoretical frameworks combined with 'practical' apprenticeship. Historically, the preclinical stage is descended from the non-vocational and humanities-based education of the physician, whereas the clinical years are a modification of the unstructured apprenticeship of the surgeon-apothecary. That is to say, the main training value of these clinical years comes largely from the results of personal contact between 'master' and 'acolyte'.

Apprenticeship — despite its humble name — is a learning process of immense sophistication and complexity. It is the best known way (perhaps the only way) to transmit high-order skills between individuals. The psychological mechanism for apprenticeship is known as 'modelling'. The conditions for modelling are that the student must respect and wish to emulate the expert — primarily in terms of knowledge and skill; but there is also an inevitable 'moral' quality which is also learned at the same time, and which contextualizes the technique (the 'medical morality', as we have called it). For this process to work there should be a voluntary suspension of critical judgement — the student recognizes that, until the apprenticeship is completed, he or she is not fully competent to criticize in any fundamental sense. There is, in effect, a two-stage process consisting, firstly, of an openness and the absorption of an ethos and a set of skills; and, secondly, of a stage when the lessons have been learned and the newly educated doctor can introduce a personal angle following on from criticism and reflection.

It is therefore vital that an apprenticeship is sufficiently long-lasting to allow effective modelling, but not so long as to destroy irreversibly the capacity for criticism and reflection. It is between these two rocks that medical education must navigate. Another more obvious dilemma is the tension between length of apprenticeship and range of coverage.

8.3   Books or lectures?

Before commencing our discussion of the apprenticeship elements, we should consider how best to cover the theoretical aspects of clinical medicine. Of course, such theoretical aspects are discussed, formally and casually, as a part of bedside teaching; but there is a further need for extensive and *systematic* coverage which must be met by reading, supplemented, to a varying extent, by lectures.

It is obvious that the only good lecture is a good lecture (in other words, bad lectures are a damaging waste of time); having said that, we note that there are a vast number of functions which a lecture can fulfil, such as providing an introduction to a topic or an explanation of a problem; distilling research findings; conveying enthusiasm; and, of course, having an amusement value. This is even more the case for a *series* of lectures; and a series of lectures by a series of people adds yet a further dimension. In a nutshell, the clinical lectures, *en masse*, can present the distinctive traditions of a medical school. They can act as a powerful form of social glue to reinforce the class identity established during the preclinical years, and they allow all these students to experience the 'wit and wisdom' of the major consultants, lecturers, and professors of their medical school. They function, therefore, to amplify the apprenticeship element in a communal sense: the apprenticeship of *a class* of students to a *faculty* of medical educators.

Such considerations should not be underestimated. Nevertheless, some students will always prefer to study privately using books. This method has the great advantage of inculcating a habit of self-education which will serve the doctor well throughout a long career away from the influence of the medical school. Private study also enables the student to focus upon areas of particular interest, and perhaps to pursue questions beyond the sheltered waters of textbooks and into the uncharted seas of original papers published in scholarly journals . . .

The blend of formal lectures and private study is highly variable in different medical schools, which is as it should be. Some schools also have the advantage of good textbooks (or desktop-published handouts) written by their own staff, which produce some of the distinctive and local qualities of lecture courses in a more portable form. But whatever the mixture of theoretical and practical which obtains, it would seem wise to aim for a combination of the benefits of both aspects of study; books *and* lectures.

8.4   Hospitals versus community

It is largely a historical accident that medical education currently happens in or around hospitals. Up until the eighteenth (or even nineteenth) century the apprentice surgeon or apothecary would train wherever his master happened to practise — whether town or country; while physicians were often educated at universities lacking any link with a hospital. This was a perfectly rational basis for medical education at the time: doctors were trained in the same kind of environment in which they intended to work, on the time-honoured basis that service is the best education.

The forces which brought medical training into the hospitals were various. As centralized and systematic education became established and prestigious, it was common for an ambitious student to supplement the apprenticeship (or his university degree) with courses of lectures at cities such as London and Edinburgh. Such courses might be at a university or at a private 'extra-mural' college; but wherever they were located, the key subject of that era was anatomy. And in those pre-embalming days, anatomy implied access to hospitals to procure the necessary fresh cadavers. Surgeons in particular regarded good practice as based on the scientific principles of anatomy, and it was this which brought surgical apprentices into the hospitals; nevertheless, the subject was seen as fundamental to all branches of medicine — and beyond (we read of philosophers, theologians, and other men of learning and culture attending dissections as part of their general education!)

After medical students had become attached to hospitals for the purposes of anatomical/surgical training there developed the familiar centralized educational scheme, with surgical 'dressers' and medical 'clerks' engaged in 'walking the wards' to imbibe the manners and mores of the great Victorian consultants. This reached its highest development in London, where education was not based in a university, but in those ancient charitable institutions, the teaching hospitals. From here it was but a small step to reach our present arrangements.

Seen in this perspective we can explain the strange paradox that clinical medical education is mostly a matter of hospital-based consultants training students to become community-based general practitioners. It is also worth noting that until the 1970s hospital-trained graduates — probably with no experience of general practice whatsoever — could set up as GP principals on the day they obtained full registration. (Even today, trainees are only required to spend one year in a general practice as part of a vocational scheme.) These almost accidental causes behind hospital-based education are worth remembering when consultants challenge the inclusion of general-practice attachments as a major component of clinical training. On the contrary, it is a perfectly sensible example of the principle that the best possible training for a career is an apprenticeship with someone doing the job for which you wish to be trained. Professor McCormick has more to say on this subject in Chapter 11.

Anyway, the situation in which we find ourselves, whatever its advantages and disadvantages, has the virtue of being our starting-point, and one which 'does the job'. So that, although it would be a rational alternative to set up from scratch a system of clinical medical education that was based upon primary care and took place mostly in general practice (as has, indeed, happened in other countries around the world), it is not likely — and probably not desirable — that the highly evolved and sophisticated British system should switch to such an arrangement at this late date.

8.5   Which specialties?

If we accept that the British way of medical education is now, and is likely to remain, one based upon hospital teaching, we should consider which specialties ought to be included, and what weight should be given to each. To answer this is not straightforward, and depends upon what is perceived to be the purpose or goal of clinical undergraduate education.

It is a truism in educational and administrative circles that the undergraduate clinical period should be regarded as a part of basic medical education. So that its aim is *not* to produce a 'safe general practitioner' ready to practise on the day of graduation, but instead to produce a general-purpose, pluripotential doctor for further training as a pre-registration house officer and then in one of the vocational schemes. In other words 'We are all specialists now.' However, despite the explicit nature of this goal, this is not how things are perceived either by the student or by the majority of the medical profession, which regards the principal aim of clinical education as the provision of useful house officers who require the minimum of supervision and training. Considering the deeply unsatisfactory nature of the pre-registration year (discussed below), we hold that this latter goal is too limited, and conflicts sharply with the long-term goals of education for a lifetime of medical practice.

Even if we accept a long-term view of the purpose of clinical undergraduate education it remains far from clear exactly which subjects students should study. Of all the British doctors who practise, about half are destined to become general practitioners, while the other half are divided between consultant specialties, of which the largest are anaesthetics, psychiatry, the various branches of medicine and surgery, obstetrics and gynaecology, and the many distinct types of laboratory-based specialty. These 'major' specialties could reasonably be regarded as providing a 'core curriculum' of subjects which the student should experience: they are, statistically speaking, the most likely directions for future specialization. But even here there are problems when the multitude of virtually independent branches of each specialty are considered. Medical practice in a highly evolved health service is so fragmented that there is no possibility of students' spending a useful amount of time in all branches of the subject. We are forced to consider what might amount to *core skills* in medicine, and how such attributes might best be attained.

On reflection there seem to be quite a number of core clinical skills to do with the whole business of meeting patients and 'taking a history'; fewer to do with physical examination (procedures such as taking a pulse and blood pressure, auscultation, and feeling an abdomen); and even fewer to do with essential knowledge for management. There is also the vital, but nebulous 'medical morality' to be absorbed (see above). Any requirement for 'pathological' or 'laboratory' knowledge is highly variable between specialties.

Our difficulties are compounded by the fact that it is hard to justify the present privileged positions of general medicine and general surgery — culminating in their duopoly of the pre-registration year. It is now the case that 'general' medicine and 'general' surgery no longer exist except in inaccessible communities and underdeveloped countries. Owing to the rising standards of expectations, these subjects are now finely subdivided into the medicine of the various systems and age-groups, and the surgery of the various bits of the body. It is hard to see why the experience of a student on a diabetic medical ward should *necessarily* count as more 'general' than that of a student in a psychiatric admissions ward, or doing the job of a casualty officer, or even working with an anaesthetist (including some involvement with intensive therapy) in a district hospital.

We do not intend to imply that the 'minor' specialties are minor in any other sense than that they employ relatively few consultants. On the contrary, paediatric and dermatological knowledge, for example, is vital to all general practitioners; and the kind of training obtained in, say, neurology or urology is every bit as valuable from the point of view of 'core skills' as that obtained in 'general' medicine or surgery. However, on the one hand, it seems reasonable that all doctors in a unified profession with a single 'portal of entry' (i.e. the MB degree or its equivalent) should have some common core of shared *experience* as well as skill; while, on the other hand, exactly because dermatology and paediatrics are a large part of general practice, they are eminently teachable to that level by a general practitioner. The same applies to the recognition for referral of neurological disease in hospital specialties — this can be taught by doctors outside the specialty.

In the final analysis, the GP or consultant is responsible for the *management* of only a restricted range of conditions, and the remainder of medicine is largely a question of *recognition* and *referral*. This kind of wisdom — when and how to treat, when to refer — may be obtained by a highly variable blend of experience; but the most important experience is inevitably at the level of apprenticeship to a specialist — in other words a GP may be the best person to teach 'urology-for-the-GP' of the type which the student intends to become. There is a significant difference between training to *be* a specialist and training someone *about* a specialty — the first can only be done by a specialist, while the second may be better done by a doctor from a quite different field.

8.6   Duration of study

If, as we have argued, the essence of medicine is centred on the clinical relationship between the doctor and the patient, then the student requires contact with patients under the close instruction of qualified doctors. This can be obtained in a wide variety of clinical contexts. All that is required (given suitable conditions, and willingness on the parts of student, doctor, and patients) is sufficient *time* for learning to occur. Therefore the selection of specialties — whatever they might be, and however varied according to the traditions and excellences of each medical school — must not be so wide and various as to prevent the time necessary for a satisfactory apprenticeship relationship to develop.

One of the interesting aspects of 'bedside' teaching is that it happens at every level; all doctors will teach those with less experience than themselves, and even final-year students have useful tips to give the junior students. This 'waterfall' of knowledge, skill, and the fruits of experience helps to make the medical apprenticeship — prolonged though it is — one which has a strong sense of progression through graded stages. The 'waterfall' has evolved in a teaching hospital setting where the medical hierarchy is at its most fully developed in the shape of the phenomenon of consultant firms that produce and maintain distinctive practices, propagated through the overlapping generations of junior doctors who pass through. All this is a powerful mechanism of professionalization — but it takes time to have an effect.

In parenthesis, it must be conceded that when 'everybody' is a teacher the quality of bedside teaching is very uneven. Some doctors, for whatever reason, seem addicted to a highly aggressive style of confrontational questioning which is designed to assert their own superiority while exposing the student's lack of knowledge in the most humiliating fashion possible. However, this may be part of the price we pay for such a high volume of (mostly) unpaid instruction. Not every doctor is a gifted teacher; but enough of them are to ensure that the student is given at least the chance to learn from several clinicians worthy of 'respect'.

It is important to emphasize that if we wish such a process of professionalization to continue (and the authors of this book are in general enthusiastic about the potential benefits of professionalization) then we must ensure that the desirability for *range* of coverage — each student getting a 'taste' of each specialty — must not be allowed to detract from the *time* available to build up a personal ('master–apprentice') relationship between the student and at least one good doctor (preferably a consultant). This is one minimum requirement for clinical medical *education*, as opposed to training in the knowledge and skills of practice.

If we accept that some kind of rotation through some combination of the above-mentioned half-dozen 'major' hospital
specialties (perhaps medicine, paediatrics, surgery, anaesthetics,
psychiatry, and obstetrics and gynaecology) plus an attachment
to general practice is a good basis for clinical education, then
we are left with a choice of what to do about the 'little' subjects (or subspecialties), such as venereology, neurology, dermatology, urology, neurosurgery, psychotherapy, etc. Here
we have a choice. These can either be given in a multitude
of 'taster' courses, perhaps just as lecture/demonstrations —
accepting that no deep understanding, of the apprentice type,
can be expected from such an approach; or else they can be
made the subject of *options*, which allow fewer of them to be
studied, but to a greater depth. There are advantages to each
approach.

However, the curricular pressure in an evolving health
service is always towards a multiplication of short attachments
of a week or two, so that no professional sub-groups are 'left
out', to help with future recruitment to the minor specialties,
and so that the particular expertise of the specialist may be
transmitted to the student. It is worth remembering that —
valid as these reasons are — there is another side to the question, and that there is a considerable price to pay for giving
every department a piece of the curriculum. Coverage by direct
experience is desirable but not essential, and it must never be
allowed to interfere with the truly essential part of clinical
education: the apprenticeship.

8.7   The pre-registration year

Moving onwards through the doctor's educational life we now
come to another 'black spot' and disaster area: the pre-
registration year, also known as the house year, the residency
(in Scotland), and the internship (in the USA). This lies at
the end of undergraduate medical education rather as an
assault course might, sadistically, be placed at the end of a
forced march! Perhaps nowhere else in medicine do we see
such a mismatch between educational ideals and the cynicism
of actual practice. Nevertheless, the pre-registration year was
introduced in 1951 explicitly for educational reasons; and

despite these reasons' having been 'hijacked' by service considerations, it is worth considering what kind of job the residency ought to be, compared with what it is. In Chapter 9 Dr Calman will consider specific and focused questions relating to the education of house-officers; here we will make points of a more general nature.

The problem of matching education and service has been that the service commitment has expanded to produce a situation where the house officer is often the *single most important* member of the firm. By 'important' is meant that if the intern is off sick, or away on holiday, then some form of locum cover must be arranged instantly; while any other member of the hierarchy (up to, and even especially, the consultant) can be covered by other members of the team. This indispensability is related, not to unique skill or ability, but to hours of work and job demarcations: in other words to the fact that house officers are actually present in the hospital for most of the time, and prepared to do almost anything.

Those specialties within which house officers' positions are located are — in the vast majority of cases — surgical and medical; although a smattering of obstetrics and gynaecology and general practice jobs are also available in some centres. The avowed purpose of the pre-registration year is quite simple: it is the final stage in a doctor's general apprenticeship before specialist training, and a completion of those 'core skills' regarded as essential for all registered doctors. Thus it is the *content* of the job, and not the nature of its specialty, which is important; and the conditions must be present for learning by apprenticeship. On the house officer's side, there should be respect and keenness to learn; on the supervising doctor's side, there should be concern for the resident's best interests — a concern to educate and not to exploit.

8.8 Objectives for improvement

Attempts to improve the educational content of house jobs fall into the positive and the negative: what house officers should do, and what they shouldn't. On the positive side it is uncontroversial that the year should build confidence by a process of graded and supervised increase in responsibility.

There should be an improvement in the core clinical skills such as general communication, specific history-taking, examination, investigation, and management (including the business of running a ward). Furthermore, the fledgeling doctor should establish the habit of actively seeking out continuing education, in contrast to the more passive and receptive habits of undergraduate life. Such continuing education is one part of a process of self-appraisal (informal and perhaps formal) by which performance is monitored and improved.

Such excellent objectives are defeated by a cavalier lack of respect combined with relentless pressure of work and excessive hours. If we use an analogy with behaviour therapy: learning to cope with the fear of clinical responsibility should come from a *graded* exposure to stressful clinical situations, rather than the make-or-break technique of 'flooding' with maximum stress. Even the maxim 'see one, do one, teach one' often seems less like cynicism and more like a counsel of perfection — and 'do one blindly (mess it up), then another, and then another . . . until you get it right' is a slogan apparently closer to the reality. There is often a *macho* attitude to medical practice which is destructive of education: a pretence that 'in at the deep end' is actually good for the doctor (if not for the patient, who may be less happy to act as a disposable experimental animal). The resulting acute stress — whereby tired and harassed house officers find themselves thrown into situations beyond their competence, in serious danger of harming the patients, but discouraged by the prevailing 'gung ho' spirit from asking for help — while perhaps acting as a crude and cheap technique for increasing confidence, might also seem specifically designed to inculcate callous and selfish attitudes.

The authors are aware of a situation in which a house officer from another country turned up for his first day and first job to find a ward empty of doctors (they were in theatre all day), a stack of patients waiting to be clerked for an unfamiliar specialty, and an even bigger stack of urgent investigations to be done. The resident, in a state of considerable nervousness, and with no available help, had great difficulty obtaining blood samples; the work continued to pile up; and the situation rapidly got out of control. After two days the unfortunate intern bolted in panic and was never seen again. It is difficult to know how typical this story is; but the point is that it happened, not in a state of emergency, but as a result of the *normal* technique for inducting house officers. It is hardly surprising that the rate of parasuicide, anecdotally, seems strikingly high during the pre-registration year; and 'self-destructive' patterns of drinking alcohol seem almost the norm.

The point of retailing the above 'horror story' is to emphasize that frequently no provision whatever is made for the newly arrived house officer, who is simply expected to clock in and do the job. No member of staff is detailed to instruct them — no member of staff is even given the time to do so; work is expected to carry on as usual, and it is a case of sink or swim — and any deficiency is blamed on the resident. But even when house officers are robust and competent, and their introduction is more helpful and humane, the system invariably results in a bad deal for the patients — doctors like to joke that you should never get ill on the first of August or February. The fact that this situation of seriously sub-standard clinical service is blandly accepted is inexcusable. New residents face *predictable* difficulties; and it should not be beyond the wit of senior medical staff to ensure that, for the first few days at least, they are given a high degree of supervision and training around the clock — both so that they can learn their jobs properly, and also so that the public are treated properly.

8.9   What is the job?

The house officers' difficulties in learning medicine are multiplied by the common situation in which they are expected to spend most of their time doing other things entirely. The University of London has laid down a set of guidelines of *inappropriate* duties for house officers, which is very revealing of the kinds of things they are increasingly being expected to do as a matter of routine: acting as admissions officers, porters, ward clerks, and phlebotomists: and performing routine intravenous injections of antibiotics, cytotoxic drugs, contrast media, etc. The report also lays down minimum standards for staff residences (there is a lively fund of anecdotes circulating among locum house officers about the range of conditions actually met with — including no food available, no baths or showers, and paper sheets on the beds!). London University's seemingly very modest range of minimum requirements are typically regarded by recently registered doctors as pie-in-the-sky; ruling out, as they do, virtually every existing house officer's position in Britain!

There is a vast and growing literature on the problem of long hours for junior doctors; and, while this problem is not confined to the pre-registration year, the situation is perhaps most severe during this time. The consensus — both in the medical profession and among the broader public — is that the present working hours are too long for education, for safety, and for humanity (there are, however, some groups of clinicians — particularly surgeons — who regard the present situation as necessary for adequate training; even a few who feel that present hours are insufficient for the requisite breadth and depth of experience). What is interesting about the question of long hours is that the situation has been allowed to persist for so long without massive protest or change. Presumably there are both positive and negative reasons. The negative reason is obvious enough: cheap labour. The positive reason is also obvious when listening to informal conversations between doctors, although it seldom reaches print. It is that the pre-registration year is a kind of initiation into medicine, a test to see if new doctors have 'the right stuff', if they are tough enough for a gruelling job; and if they have none of these qualities to begin with, then by the end they should have been licked into shape, stripped of their namby-pamby idealism, toughened in nerve and sinew, and brought into line with the rest of the profession. That last point gives the key: the house job is seen as a swift, and perhaps brutal, but efficient mechanism of professionalization.

But is it a good thing? Does it make people better doctors? Well, such questions are notoriously vague and difficult to answer. On the one hand, there is little doubt that confidence and competence are radically transformed during the pre-registration year, and to that extent it must be counted a success. On the other hand, there is an equally obvious coarsening of attitude among many or most young doctors as a result of their experience: it is here more than anywhere that the infamous qualities of medical arrogance and insensitivity take root and flourish. Furthermore, far from the year's laying the foundations for a lifetime's continuing medical education, house officers are notorious for never opening a book from one end of the year to the other. It takes a major effort to resume studying for professional qualifications after the habit has been so decisively broken.

8.10   A declining prospect?

All of this would not be so bad if there were a perception that things were improving; but this does not seem to be the case. The administrative load is probably increasing with each passing year, and house officers are at the front line when it comes to patching up the deficiencies of a health service which is — in parts — on the verge of collapse. The various professional groups may battle it out for diminishing resources; but so far as the resident is concerned 'the buck stops here'. All too often the interns feel themselves to be mere pawns in the quasi-political games played by other more powerful groups, with every increase in bureaucratization rebounding on them. At the point of interface of acute medical care with the public, on a round-the-clock basis, these inexperienced and overworked staff are faced with the most difficult choices, with the 'responsibility' for potentially disastrous consequences landing squarely on their shoulders. In such a situation it is clear that house officers feel both exploited and undervalued — nobody would seem to want their advice or opinions on what the real problems of the health service are from the point of view of those doing most of the work in it.

In addition to the escalating stresses of service there is an objective decline in conditions. The facilities available to the resident medical staff have proved an attractive target for hospital administrators under powerful pressure to save money. The detailed recommendations for accommodation from the University of London are a response to the progressive erosion of the standard of rooms and of the availability of food and amenities for 'rest and recreation'. To some extent the decline in conditions is simply disruptive of the doctor's comfort and convenience: but its real importance is more that it is symbolic of an utter disregard of residents' well-being.

8.11   Educational possibilities

The educational problems, not to mention the wider issues, associated with the pre-registration year are — to say the least — formidable. They are formidable to the point that the most reasonable option might be to forget any pretence that the pre-registration year is educational at all; and to accept that it is purely a period of exploitive 'scut work' for the unfortunate 'house dog' — something to be endured with as much avoidance of pain possible. There is little doubt concerning the depth of demoralization among residents, who are sceptical about the likelihood of significant improvement, and who therefore adopt a policy of damage-limitation.

However true this may be, the authors are committed to the improvement of medical education, broadly within the boundaries of current organizational practice. Given that the year is so difficult, and that things are not likely to change rapidly, it becomes essential to ask how we can prepare students for the rigours of this period in as efficient a way as possible without losing the long-term and educational aspects of the undergraduate clinical curriculum. Some progress has been made in this direction by focusing upon the 'critical incidents' of the year in an attempt to locate the key skills or experiences required, as Dr Calman describes in Chapter 9.

Deficiencies in these identified key areas may be addressed during the undergraduate years, although there is a sense in which even the best theoretical preparation is likely to prove inadequate in the unpredictable and fraught situations of actual practice. The most useful strategy is the actual *presence* (not just the availability at the end of a telephone) of an experienced doctor to act as a guide and friend. It is worth emphasizing, at this point, that the most vital relationship for a house officer at the day-to-day level is the one with his or her immediate superior: the senior house officer or registrar. It is the quality of this association which determines much of the value (or misery) of the pre-registration year. Personal likes and dislikes are, of course, unpredictable; but the conditions for a healthy working relationship can be optimized by having time set aside at the very beginning of the job for the formal, detailed, and personal induction of a new doctor.

This said, the consultant's role must not be underestimated. This is comprehensive, ranging as it does from the establishment of a general ward atmosphere and manner of practice, to the task of providing a 'reference' for the junior doctors to obtain other jobs. The vexed question of references is at the heart of much frustration. Doctors' future careers are understood to be at the mercy of their bosses' opinions. This is one major factor which seems to underlie the frequent problems in communication between the different grades: it is considered unwise to admit to mistakes, lack of confidence, or deficiencies in competence; or to complain about conditions — nobody wishes to be known as a whinger . . . In a competitive world (in competition even with one's house officer colleagues) anger and frustration are dissipated in moaning to unthreatening friends and relations — or just kept to oneself.

The pre-registration year is a situation as near to unremitting gloom as we find in medical education — not least because it is a scandal in terms of simple human equity. Nevertheless, it is unconstructive to give up in despair. Efforts must be unremitting to improve the lot of the house officer; and the educational perspective offers us a powerful lever for change, as it is here that high-minded official intentions and the squalor of actual practice are most indefensibly at odds.

8.12 Conclusions

1. The clinical years of undergraduate education, based on 'apprenticeship' supplemented by systematic teaching, seem reasonably well-designed. However, the requirement for a broad factual coverage must not be allowed to swamp the educational objectives, as seems to have happened with Mr J.

2. The pre-registration year is open to serious criticism, and represents the worst of medical educational practice.

Bibliography

Calman, K. C., Fraser, J., Harden, R. M., and Murray, C. (1986). Educational objectives of the pre-registration year. *Medical Teacher*, 8, 383–7.

General Medical Council (1980). *Recommendations on basic medical education*. GMC, London.

Lawrence, C. (1988). Alexander Monro *primus* and the Edinburgh manner of anatomy. *Bulletin of the History of Medicine*, **62**, 193–214.

Oakeshott, M. (1962). *Rationalism in politics and other essays*. Methuen, London.

University of London (1991). Inappropriate duties for preregistration house officers. *British Medical Journal*, **302**, opposite p. 571.

9 The pre-registration year
K. C. Calman

9.1 Introduction

'There has been enthusiastic support among our witnesses, including the representatives of medical schools, for the proposal that, in future, entry into independent medical practice should be preceded by a period of approved and responsible clinical practice under supervision.' Thus began the section of the Goodenough Report of 1944 on pre-registration house officers — and a long series of efforts to improve general clinical training, as the period is officially called. House officer posts were first introduced in 1951; and since that time the year has been the subject of numerous reviews, reports, and research exercises.

An analysis of the wording of this paragraph is interesting. It recommended that there should be approved posts, where it would be possible to practise medicine responsibly, and to be fully supervised in the process. These three features remain at the heart of the year, and have been reiterated in almost all subsequent documents. Yet they are areas where difficulties remain, and the most recent discussion papers from the GMC emphasize them again.

In general terms, while these principles remain, the concept that independent medical practice might be achieved by a further year of training has, of course, been superseded. In all areas of clinical practice much more experience is required. It is of interest therefore to note similar developments in other professional groups related to medicine. In some recent reports it has been suggested that in medicine the period of training at this level might be extended to two years before full registration, and the debate on this continues. In addition the changes proposed to the undergraduate curriculum, by increasing its flexibility and defining a core group of subjects, will inevitably have spin-offs for the pre-registration period of training.

At present, however, it is well recognized that all is not well. House officers work long hours; they are often poorly supervised; and the objectives of the period of training are unclear. There is little or no time for educational activities; and they may not even be encouraged. During this period many attitudes and habits are set, and the process of indoctrination or initiation, the hidden agenda of medical practice, takes place. Yet it should be a time of excitement, learning, and growth. Perhaps one of the difficulties is that while the objectives have been stated many times they are generally not known by the house officers, and not 'owned' by the senior staff. It is relevant therefore to discuss what the aims and objectives might be, before developing ways in which the period of training might be improved.

9.2   The general aims

These might be (Calman *et al.* 1986):

(1)   to continue the process of basic medical education; and

(2)   to afford the graduate balanced clinical experience and increasing responsibility for the care of patients

The experience gained in the year should help the young doctor to:

(a)   *Develop confidence.* The training under supervision should allow confidence to grow. Making decisions, and talking to patients, relatives, and others are integral parts of this process.

(b)   *Accept responsibility.* As experience increases the opportunity occurs to take decisions on the investigation, management, and care of patients, and to accept the responsibility for these decisions, which also implies an acknowledgement of the ethical issues involved in decision-making.

(c)   *Improve communication skills.* This is an essential part of learning, and, if not developed properly at this stage, can affect clinical competence later.

(d)   *Acquire practical skills.* The importance of history-taking clinical examination, and the appropriate use of investigations should become clear. The cost of these to individual patients and in financial terms should also become clear.

(e)   *Work as part of a team.* This includes the work of the ward unit team — the consultants, registrars, nurses, domestics, and members of other health care professions; and the extended team — general practitioners, health visitors, community nurses, dietitians, etc.

(f) *Realize the importance of continuing medical education.* Young doctors must be aware of the importance of self-education, so that they may continue to extend their knowledge skills and attitudes throughout their professional career.

(g) *Assess progress and performance.* The interaction between consultant and house officer is crucial to success, as is the degree of supervision. Feedback to the doctor about his or her performance is important in establishing standards of clinical practice.

9.3 Objectives of the pre-registration year

These general aims can be developed further into more specific objectives that describe what the doctor should be able to do at the end of the period of training. These objectives would comprise:

A. acquiring a knowledge of:

(1) disease processes and their treatment, particularly of the more common disabling diseases and those that endanger life or have serious consequences;

(2) human relationships, both personal and social, and the interaction between patients and their physical and social environment;

(3) emergencies and how to deal with them;

(4) the amelioration of suffering and disability;

(5) rehabilitation;

(6) the organization and provision of health care delivery, and the resource consequences of decision-making; and

(7) ethical standards and responsibilities; and

B. acquiring the skills to do the following:

(1) diagnose and investigate common medical problems;

(2) manage acute medical emergencies, and the pre- and post-operative care of patients;

(3) elicit, record, and interpret symptoms and signs;

(4) identify problems and take decisions on their management;

(5)   assess the reliability of evidence and the relevance of scientific knowledge, reach conclusions by logical deduction, and evaluate critically methods and standards of clinical practice;

(6)   carry out simple practical clinical procedures;

(7)   show confidence and increasing maturity in dealing with patients and families, and demonstrate communication skills;

(8)   communicate clinical information accurately and concisely by word of mouth and in writing to medical colleagues and other professionals involved in the care of patients;

(9)   use laboratory and other diagnostic services effectively and economically; and

(10) manage time effectively and manage the workload; and

C. developing attitudes of:

(1)   caring and concern for patients and their families and for colleagues;

(2)   self-motivated learning; and

(3)   concern for ethical principles and the value-base for medical practice.

It may seem inappropriate to list these factors in such detail; but this has been done deliberately, in order to illustrate several important and general points which apply equally to other stages of clinical education. The first is the value of writing down such aims and objectives. They provide the basis, however crude, for the interaction between the consultant and the young doctor. The second reason is that they also provide some form of standard against which performance can be judged, and provide a check-list of areas to be covered. They further provide a means of checking on the supervision given to the house officer; and in the approval of posts they can provide a framework for a dialogue between the parties concerned. They also serve to point up the fact that to ensure that these aims and objectives are achieved the process needs to be managed, and there has to be a designated consultant who is responsible for any action required.

9.4   Assessment of progress

Discussion of aims and objectives and their achievement raises another issue which is also relevant to other stages of education: that of the methods involved in the assessment of progress. Perhaps the first step is to agree the objectives, and to ensure that the trainee is aware of what is expected. The second stage is to use these objectives to assess the competence of the house officer at regular intervals. This may require that the views of others (nurses, patients, other staff) are taken into account. Feedback, given in an honest and constructive way, is essential. Finally there is the need to identify areas for improvement, and to review these again at some later stage. These methods are not new, or sophisticated. They have been at the root of medical education for generations, and have always been the essence of the clinical apprenticeship system. But ask any young doctors how often they are used, and the answer will often reveal that this key part of the educational process is missing. This in itself explains much of the disgruntlement with the pre-registration year — the simple lack of feedback, supervision, and interest from senior staff. Progress in improving the outcome of medical education may not have to rely on new technology and computers, but on the application of common-sense principles.

9.5 Critical incidents

But what is the evidence that this period of training is failing to provide the education experience that it should? One set of data on this subject was collected by means of a critical incidents study of 200 house officers in the West of Scotland (Calman and Donaldson 1991). (Critical incidents are those parts of a job where intervention is clearly effective and important for diagnosis or management see Chapter 6.5.) Over 300 incidents were recorded; and when they were analysed and grouped together several main issues emerged. The largest category of incident related to personal aspects of the period of training. This fact is particularly illuminating, as it demonstrates the degree of personal involvement and the need for supervision. Many house officers were not being listened to, and felt they were being left to do things without support. It should be emphasized that this was *not* because there were no superiors available, but because consultant involvement was superficial and technical. Very few house officers seemed to be told how they were progressing, and whether they were doing well or badly. Further analysis showed that some were deficient in clinical skills and knowledge and experience of practical procedures. By the end of the year they were all fully trained; but their early months could have been much easier if they had received appropriate training in the undergraduate part of the course. In a similar way house officers would have benefited from having some training in management and the organization of work, in communication skills, and in setting priorities.

The value of such exercises is that they provide a method of identifying educational needs which can then be taken further in the appropriate part of the continuum of medical education. The information should not only be used as a criticism of some preceding part of the process, but as a positive way of improving the experience provided. This illustration also provides a clear example of the role of educational research in improving the quality of training, whose results should in turn be seen in benefits to patients and to the outcomes of health care — the real end-point of medical education.

A review of the wider literature in this field reveals other problems (Alexander *et al.* 1985; Deary and Tait 1987; Firth-Cozens 1987; Leslie *et al.* 1990). The long hours on duty, and the effect they might have on performance, are regularly noted. In addition there have been comments on stress and emotional distress, which can lead to errors of judgement. Much of this has been related to the Libby Zion case, in which long hours worked resulted in clinical errors (Asch and Parker 1988). There also appears to be a clearly defined 'pre-residency syndrome', which is associated with the anxiety that occurs in senior medical students before they take up their first hospital appointments (Swanson 1985).

Each of these studies illustrates the problems associated with the year. Yet they may appear to identify only the negative aspects; while in fact a very positive rise in confidence and maturity, and in the ability to take decisions and accept responsibility are also apparent. The key is to marry extensive clinical experience with educational opportunities. How this might be done will be the subject of the final part of this chapter. Before approaching this topic, however, two further matters need first to be considered.

9.6 The need for supervised training

The first is the general issue of the need, or otherwise, for a period of training at this time, under supervision, before full registration and independent practice is permitted. This, stated in another way, raises the general question as to what experience is required to become competent, and how this is to be measured. Such an issue is also relevant to other professional groups, and is in no sense peculiar to medicine. Few would dispute that the undergraduate course requires to be supplemented by further experience, and that this experience should be supervised and assessable. For many of the specialties, if not all of them, the pre-registration year is but the first hurdle, and in no sense constitutes the end of training. But addressing this topic does raise the question as to how long the pre-registration period should be. Arguments have been put forward over the years for lengthening it to two years; and no doubt the debate on this will continue. Perhaps this aspect is less important than the need to have an effective clinical year followed by a period of postgraduate training in a particular specialty, coupled with a recognition of the importance of entering upon a lifelong process of continuing education.

The second issue relates to the range and type of experience provided during the year. In general this has been in general medicine and surgery, with or without a short period in a specialty. In a very small number of cases a six-month period in general practice has been available. This has been noted to be of considerable value, but is difficult to arrange (Harris 1986). In defining the posts, it is necessary to assess their educational value, and the quality of the supervision associated with them. Those who have the responsibility for this should be both innovative in the range of posts covered and active in ensuring quality.

9.7 Clinical experience and educational opportunity

The first is the need to set overall objectives for the period of training. This requires clarity in the overall vision for the training of the doctor, and a clear view as to the 'kind' of doctor that will result from the training. These arguments have been rehearsed in another part of the book. In specific terms, however, the objectives for any part of the course must be informed both by the nature of the preceding period (in this case the undergraduate course) and by the future direction for the individual (in this case very variable). Further, the objectives have to be practical, and related to the clinical practice of the doctor. Relevance is therefore crucial. In this instance the critical incidents study has revealed a number of areas for improvement.

Besides defining the objectives, they have to be communicated to all concerned. Without this, lists of closely written prose worked on by great educational minds will not be used. In general those who need to see, and agree, objectives are the house officer and the consultant supervisor. However, the net is in practice much wider than this, and must include the rest of the clinical team, nurses in particular, and those who manage the service. Without such wider discussion the relevance of the objectives, and of their subsequent implementation, is unlikely to be recognized.

The second issue relates to supervision. As has been noted in other sections of this book, the apprenticeship system is often an appropriate model for medical education. In such a context those functioning as the 'masters' in the master–apprentice relationship carry a number of responsibilities. At the most basic level this implies a degree of concern for ensuring that the maximum opportunities are taken to impart and acquire educational experiences. Further, there is a need to provide direct and honest feedback on performance. This is critical, and is associated with the concept of competence — a difficult and challenging educational idea. From the critical incident study it is clear that currently feedback is deficient, and anecdotal evidence would suggest that such a situation is not unique to the pre-registration year. Yet unless the consultant staff take this aspect of their work seriously, the benefits of the relationship will be lost.

This takes us to the third issue, that of monitoring and evaluating education programmes. How should it be done, how often should a formal review be instituted, and what action should be taken if performance is not up to scratch? For the year under review, it has been suggested that on two or three occasions in each six-month period a formal interview should take place, during which objectives and performance are reviewed. During these times there will be an opportunity for the parties to get to know each other and to form the beginnings of the long-lasting professional relationship that is the heart of the apprenticeship system. As a part of this process new objectives are also set for subsequent review.

It is also clear that the objectives for any period of training must not be developed in 'medical' terms alone. While medical skill and expertise, together with the ability to carry out practical procedures, are clearly important, other aspects must also be considered. These could well include communication skills and the abilities to organize personal time, to set priorities, and to manage resources. There is also the need for the house officer to develop skills in taking decisions, and to understand the ethical implications of those decisions.

Finally, any period of training must reinforce the concept of continuing education. While it is particularly difficult to have formal educational programmes during the year, this does not exempt the individual, encouraged by the consultant, from engaging in a lifelong process of self-education. This topic will be taken up further in subsequent sections of this book.

9.8 Conclusions

The period of pre-registration training presents a microcosm of medical training as a whole and though it has its own particular problems it can be used as a model to test general educational principles.

Bibliography

Alexander, D., Monk, J. S., and Jonas, A. P. (1985). Occupational stress, personal strain and coping among residents and faculty members. *Journal of Medical Education*, **60**, 830–9.

Asch, D. A., and Parker, R. M. (1988). The Libby Zion case: one step forwards or two steps backward? *New England Journal of Medicine*, **318**, 771–5.

Calman, K. C., and Donaldson, M. (1991). The pre-registration house-officer year: a critical incident study. *Medical Education*, **25**, 51–9.

Calman, K. C., Fraser, J., Harden, R. M., and Murray, C. (1986). Educational objectives of the pre-registration year. *Medical Teacher*, **8**, 383–7.

Deary, I. J., and Tait, R. (1987). Effects of sleep disruption on cognitive performance and mood in medical house officers. *British Medical Journal*, **295**, 1513–16.

Firth-Cozens, J. (1987). Emotional distress in junior house officers. *British Medical Journal*, **295**, 533–6.

Harris, C. M. (1986). Pre-registration posts in general practice. *Journal of Medical Education*, **20**, 136–9.

Leslie, P. J., Williams, J. A., McKenna, C., Smith, G., and Heading, R. C. (1990). Hours, volume and type of work of pre-registration house officers. *British Medical Journal*, **300**, 1038–41.

Swanson, A. G. (1985). The 'pre-residency syndrome': an incipient epidemic of educational disruption. *Journal of Medical Education*, **60**, 201–2.

10 *Continuing medical education*
K. C. Calman

10.1 Introduction

Continuing medical education (CME) may be defined as a series of processes aimed at improving health care through learning, either by individual efforts or as part of activities organized by a provider unit. Conventionally CME begins following appointment to a substantive post as a specialist or general practitioner — that is, at the end of postgraduate or higher medical training. It is more than that of course: as has been emphasized throughout this book, education, as a lifelong process, must begin at the time of entry to the medical course, and be seen to be an attitude of mind, rather than something added on at the end of formal 'training'. While this chapter will therefore deal with the process of CME as a distinct entity, its roots in earlier parts of medical education should not be forgotten.

First, a consideration of the definition given at the start of this section. It should be noted that CME has a very definite purpose, that of improving patient care. It has therefore a very clear *raison d'être*, based on the fact that medical and scientific knowledge expand continuously and that the doctor in whatever specialty must keep up to date in knowledge, skills, and attitudes. The consequences of not doing so imply that patient care may be less than adequate, and that individual patients may not be managed appropriately. There is therefore a moral dimension to CME.

A further implication is that, in addition to improving the skills of individual doctors and the treatment provided, CME is a major agent for change in health and health care. New knowledge of treatment, new methods of delivering care, and new techniques for assessment can all be implemented if the system for CME is working effectively. There is therefore a broad and increasingly important dimension to CME — that of improving health care as a whole.

CME may be viewed as a process carried out by an individual doctor, to meet his or her own needs. This can be organized as a process of self-education, motivated by a wish to provide the best possible care to patients. It can also be organized by a series of provider units (Universities, Colleges, Specialty Groups, etc.), who provide a range of learning experiences, from which doctors can choose specific topics or courses. Most doctors use a mixture of self-directed and more formally organized learning programmes. In general it can be regarded as the end stage of the transition from institutional learning, such as occurs in most medical schools, to individual learning based on clearly defined needs.

Any consideration of CME will, of necessity, be concerned with a very wide range of issues. In this chapter we will consider how doctors learn; the settings in which they work; the ethical dimension of CME; the definition of competence and its evaluation; evidence, or otherwise, for the value of CME; quality and standards; the role of the medical audit; and the place of the medical society in CME.

10.2 How doctors learn

Even a brief examination of the topic will show that doctors learn in surprisingly diverse ways. The lecture is perhaps the first to come to mind; yet it may be the least important for the specialist, who requires very specific information from other specialists. This is not to say that lectures do not have value — they may be important in keeping a specialist up to date with topics outside his or her own field of interest — but that they are a relatively inefficient way of transmitting information. Specialist or generalist medical societies are a specialized variety of lecture audience/discussion group, and will be discussed in more detail later.

Discussion groups or seminars may be more appropriate than lectures for CME, allowing much more interaction between the facilitator of the group and the individual doctor. This is particularly the case if learning objectives are specified at the beginning, and the doctor provides input from personal experience. The value of medical audit in this process will be discussed later.

Personal observation or demonstration of new techniques is a further development of this, and is especially relevant in the surgical specialties, or where invasive procedures are to be carried out. There can, however, be no substitute for practical hands-on experience in this area. Apprenticeship is perhaps the best term for this, bringing out as it does the close relationship between the 'master' and the learner on a one-to-one basis. For the development of new skills there is a need to learn under supervision, and to be guided through the procedure. Examples of such skills which have required experienced doctors, often of some standing, to learn completely new skills include laparoscopic procedures; angioplasties; and invasive radiological techniques. The relative efficiency of this 'apprenticeship' method as an educational tool can be measured by the number of those who then practise the procedure. There is little doubt that this is a key method in CME.

A further method is by personal reading, either alone or as part of a journal club. Some evidence suggests that, contrary to popular belief, doctors do not use this method as often as might be presumed. They tend to read a limited number of journals related to their own special interests, and unless they have special research needs rarely move out of their own fields.

Journal clubs have a special place, encouraging as they do the critical analysis of the literature. Part of this issue relates to the availability of a library and access to a wide range of material. Most accrediting bodies (Colleges and Higher Training Committees) make the presence of an adequate library a prerequisite for approval of training.

Many doctors are of course kept up to date by reports in the media, printed or electronic. Television programmes, newspaper articles, magazines, all sensitize the doctor to what is going on. In some instances patients may be better informed than the professional. This is particularly the case when the patient belongs to, or is associated with, a specialist group of patients and families associated with a particular disease or illness. Publications from such organizations can be invaluable. Doctors and other professional staff must not be afraid to learn from such groups, as their experience is generally much greater than the doctor's.

Doctors also learn from other colleagues in other disciplines, by personal contact. This is one of the commonest methods of learning, and generally very efficient. A typical situation is that the doctor, faced with a particular clinical problem which is beyond his or her own experience, or for which more expert advice is required, contacts a colleague for advice. This results in an exchange of views, and practical advice is given, perhaps associated with reading material. As a result the doctor extends his or her own experience and changes his or her clinical behaviour. The key to this method of learning is for the doctor to be able to recognize his or her own limitations, and to have good access to expertise when required. For this reason methods which encourage regular informal contact between doctors can facilitate this type of exchange. Meetings, sharing coffee-breaks, and informal social events all have their place. Restrictions placed on such events indicate a very short-term approach to improving CME, and ultimately, patient care.

Finally, doctors learn by examining their own practice and by the process of medical audit — a topic which will be discussed more fully later. As part of this, working with others, teaching others, and being constantly challenged to justify action are powerful stimuli to learn and to change. The importance of teaching others personal learning should not be under-estimated; and the value of having a research interest is part of this. Doctors have a continuing responsibility to contribute to better patient care by reviewing and evaluating their own performance.

This discussion emphasizes a number of points which have long been known to those involved in adult education: namely, that it is essential that the learning is relevant, is based on personal experience, and is interactive and practical. These lessons need to be repeated and reinforced as CME grows and becomes part of a national programme to improve patient care.

10.3   Ethical implications of CME

This leads directly into a discussion of the ethical implications of CME, or more correctly, the implications of not taking part in CME programmes. Clearly doctors have a moral obligation to provide the best and most appropriate care for individual patients. This implies, however, that they have the correct skills, knowledge, and attitudes to carry this obligation through. But how up to date do they need to be? Do they need to know everything about their special area? How many journals should they read, and how many CME sessions should they attend each month or each week? How will their performance be judged? Some test of reasonableness needs to be applied to the situation, and a practical answer to the problem has to be achieved. Two conclusions, however, are clear. The first is that doctors have an obligation to keep up to date; and for this reason alone CME needs to be supported. The second is that some test of performance, or competence, is required to ensure that standards of care are appropriate, and that quality is maintained. This also raises the issue of what to do with those who do not meet the standards, and what role educational programmes have in remedying the situation.

10.4 Competence and performance review

This is an issue central to CME. It concerns standards of care and the knowledge, skills, and attitudes which doctors should possess at different periods in their career. Thus it is possible to distinguish between the house officer and the consultant in terms of performance. The assessment of competence is an important activity, and relates the performance of an individual doctor to a given set of criteria. In general it is carried out by other doctors, and is based on comparisons with the competence of others in similar specialties and grades. There is of course no reason why it should be the responsibility of doctors. Others, including nursing staff, managers, and patients, have a role in the process. Indeed it might be claimed that they might be more objective than other doctors.

The criteria on which a judgement of competence is based can be derived in a variety of ways. The simplest is to compare the activity and the outcome of care provided by an individual doctor with that provided by a range of others. These can be done by observation and by the objective measurement of evidence of activity and outcome, such as results of treatment, scrutiny of case sheets, participation in clinical trials and the results of audit. The results may be compared with those of others working in the same geographical area, or in other parts of the country, or abroad. From such experiences it becomes possible to tabulate the criteria that the competent doctor is required to meet.

Another way of developing such criteria is to use the process of critical incident analysis. Such a process analyses the results of asking large numbers of doctors in a particular category which are the areas of particular difficulty or problems, and which the areas in which good patient care is easier to deliver. From this an assessment can be made of the skills needed in those areas — the 'competencies' — which are required to deliver a proper level of service. These can then be evaluated in the individual doctor.

Once a doctor has been designated as competent, perhaps at the end of the period of postgraduate training, the next question which arises is whether or not the doctor should at regular intervals undergo periodic re-certification. In an ideal world, CME would be the way in which doctors kept up to date. For the reasons given before, this may not be sufficient in itself without some incentive to continue to learn. It is for this reason that a number of organizations in different parts of the world have used some form of re-accreditation process. In general this involves a formal assessment of workload and outcome, as previously described, on a regular basis, for example every five years. This is not the norm at present; but a number of specialist societies and colleges are discussing its implementation.

This process, however has an important implication. There is no problem if the doctor is found to be competent, and able to be re-accredited. But what if the doctor is found wanting? This is a key issue, and for many years it has been avoided. But this cannot continue. If the profession is to be self-regulating, and to retain the confidence of the public, then it must be able to tackle these difficult problems. The General Medical Council is in the process of debating the issues of performance review; and where this system has been instituted in other countries it has usually been associated with some form of remedial education process. The supervision of the process is crucial; and there is a need for a willingness to use the ultimate sanction of removing the doctor from the list of those able to practise medicine. It is perhaps surprising that this has not happened sooner, and that machinery is not readily available to tackle the problem. Recent moves, however, are encouraging, and should lead both to a greater understanding of 'competence' and its assessment, and to the practice of a higher quality of medicine.

There is little doubt that 'quality' issues and standards are topics that are being actively debated in educational circles at the present time. Defining quality is, of course, difficult, and it is subject to different interpretations. It is, however, the role of the Universities, Colleges, and educational bodies to clarify their own thoughts on this issue. In addition to considering the problem in an academic way, there is a real need for a practical outcome. One of the key concepts in the NHS reforms is the separation of the planning or purchasing function from the provision of the service. As part of this, contracts will be set between the purchaser and provider; and part of such contracts will be concerned with quality. There is therefore an urgent need to set quality standards and to devise and develop guidelines for clinical practice. This subject will be discussed in more detail under the heading of medical audit.

10.5 The value of CME

So far it has been assumed that CME is valuable, and that somehow the educational process is translated into improved outcomes for patients, or that some measure of efficiency or value for money can readily be applied to it. But what is the evidence for this? First, there is a great deal of anecdotal information, based on observation of practice. Over a period of years an individual doctor modifies his or her practice, and introduces new drugs, procedures, and methods of working. Much of this, as has been noted previously, comes from meeting other doctors, reading the literature, and attending meetings. However, it has rarely been evaluated with any rigour, and the efficiency of the process has not been adequately tested.

There have, on the other hand, been a series of studies which have asked, in a more formal way, what evidence there is of CME's being translated into better outcomes. The disappointing fact is that there is little evidence that formal programmes of CME actually change behaviour. Even more disappointing is the fact that the studies themselves have often been inadequate to allow proper conclusions to be drawn. There is of course good evidence that knowledge is increased or changed; but little that it changes behaviour. Such a pessimistic view needs qualification, however. It is difficult to carry out such studies. There is a need for pre-teaching baseline data, which may in themselves be difficult to obtain. Further, after the learning experience, the end-point of change has to be sufficiently measurable, in a relatively short time, to allow conclusions to be drawn. Finally, following the learning the doctor has to be able to return to the clinical setting and to be able to carry out the changed practice. This can be particularly difficult if the change involves the co-operation of others in the team who have not been part of the process. Indeed this may be one of the most important reasons for the failure to translate knowledge into practice. Any effect may be masked or negated by other members of the clinical team. The difficulties of carrying out evaluative educational research can be clearly seen.

Such an analysis does, however, raise important issues relating to models of continuing education. The 'educational' model is associated with learning objectives, a programme to work through, and an assessment of outcomes. This can be very effective, but may fall down because of the constraints on trying to apply new knowledge in a disparate setting. A second model is one of the social change. In this model, not only are learning objectives required, but there is a conscious attempt made to change the environment in which the new procedure is to be introduced. Once again, this too may fail unless the whole process is managed effectively. A third model is based on a problem-solving approach in which all relevant parties are brought together to tackle a common problem, or to learn a new procedure. In general this is the most effective way of ensuring change; yet it is probably the least used. Normally a member of the junior medical staff is sent on a course on his or her own, and returns to the clinical unit fired up with new knowledge and skills and ready to implement them, only to meet resistance or even hostility.

Another way of looking at the issue is to describe the processes by which medical innovations diffuse into general clinical practice. The literature in this field describes several different types of doctor. The first group are the pioneers and enthusiasts. They are likely to be at the forefront of change, and are continually innovating and developing new ideas. In general they do not change the behaviour of others, as their ideas are often seen to be too far out. Change really begins when the second group, the pace-setters, become involved. These are professional leaders, who carry real credibility and who are looked up to by the profession as a whole. In commercial jargon, they are the project champions. Once they have picked up a new idea and endorsed it and used it themselves, then others will follow. When this occurs the majority of others will follow and take up the new idea. It should be noted, however, that all this might take several years to work through. There is indeed an almost schizophrenic attitude to innovations in the medical profession. On the one hand they will not change until they consider the evidence to be 'good'; and on the other, they will take up new and unevaluated treatments with alacrity. The rationale which distinguishes these two processes is not clear. Finally, there are the laggards, who won't change, or do so so slowly that the change is imperceptible. It is this group who do not attend CME sessions, and who do not see the need for them. This is a particularly difficult group, and one which presents a particular challenge to educationalists.

CME therefore *can* be effective. But those who organize CME on a formal basis must be aware of the pitfalls and difficulties, and be prepared to evaluate the results of their efforts not only in relation to 'customer satisfaction' and knowledge gained, but on patient outcomes. This will require a level of educational sophistication and planning which is not at present universally available. The challenge, however, is an important one.

10.6   The role of medical audit

Medical audit is not a new concept, but one which has been rediscovered by the policy makers. A variety of definitions have been used; but the one which is most commonly employed is that it is a 'process of systematically and critically analysing the outcome of medical care'. This is carried out by a process of peer review, and should take into account the resources available. The process has been called medical audit, implying that this is an activity carried out by doctors. But this is clearly not the case. All health professionals are involved; and for this reason the process is perhaps more accurately referred to as clinical audit.

The definition quoted makes several important points. First, that the process is a systematic one, in which the doctor (or other health-care professional) regularly reviews the whole range of work in which he or she is involved. Second, it is a process in which the outcome is critically analysed. It is not therefore simply a collection of data for its own sake; rather it must ask questions both as to the outcome of care and as to the ways in which the care is provided. This is absolutely essential, or otherwise the clinical audit will only examine neutral questions or those for which there are easy answers. Audit is about measuring outcome and effect on patient care, and for this reason there is a need for better and more effective methods for making such measurements. Outcome research has been neglected in favour of easier process indicators. The definition also implies that the audit process should be associated with peer review and comparison with the performance of others. As has already been suggested earlier in this chapter, this may well be appropriate; but it carries with it the responsibility for dealing with doctors (or others) who do not come up to scratch. It also raises the issue, once again, of whether doctors are the only ones who can evaluate the work of other doctors. The role of other professionals and the public may need to be taken into account. A major argument for using peer review is that only in front of other doctors would doctors be prepared to be frank and to admit to standards which are not of the highest quality. This is in fact likely to be true; and the long-standing grand rounds, clinico-pathological conferences, and ward meetings show how effective this can be. There is also some concern in the profession about the use of 'League tables' which compare the results obtained in one institution with those of another. Such comparisons are likely in the first instance to be relatively crude, and not to reflect adequately the case-mix of the hospital. The key point, however, is that this is the way thinking is going, and unless the profession gets its act together soon and associates the results of medical audit with an effective educational programme (the link to CME) an important opportunity will have been lost.

But what of the process itself? In outline the process of medical audit is like many similar cyclical schemes which involve reviewing data, changing behaviour, and monitoring progress. The educational cycle or the quality cycle would be examples of this. In essence it begins with an assessment of the issue to be audited. This might involve data-collection or an analysis of existing information. This process in itself may be sufficient to modify practice. The second step is to plan the intervention or change required. This might consist of the introduction of a new procedure, or the modification of an existing one, or a clearer definition of the standards required. The third step is to implement the plan over a period of time; and this is followed by the final step, which monitors the outcome. At any stage there may be a return to the assessment or planning stage. The cycle is then repeated, the standards being regularly updated and improved. It should be stressed that the topics chosen can represent a very wide range of issues, and that the audit can be one of outcome or one of process. The cycle described above is intimately linked to the educational cycle, which assesses knowledge, skills, and attitudes, determines the changes required to improve patient care, and implements them.

The educational implications of audit should therefore be clear, and the link with basic learning processes evident. First, the data used are personal, and there needs to be a personal commitment to clear the process. Audit is practical, in that it deals with real issues, and is therefore relevant. It is also of a problem-solving nature, and the outcome should be of direct benefit to patient care. Thus, though medical audit is only one tool in improving CME, it is a particularly powerful one because of its theoretical and practical base. It inevitably leads to discussions of quality, standards, and value for money. To be really effective it must consider resource implications; and as more and more doctors become involved in management issues it provides a professional means by which quality can be assured.

This leads to a discussion of the use of guidelines, standards, and protocols in the improvement of patient care. In general it would appear to be a good idea to ensure that methods of patient-management are written down and agreed. The educational value of doing this is, in fact, considerable. There are, however, some problems. The first is the obvious one of the patient who does not quite fit into a particular 'protocol', or who for perfectly good reasons does not wish to undergo the proposed course of management. The second is the issue of clinical freedom (if it still exists), and the need to be able to improve treatment and to have the ability to carry out research and development. The third objection is in some ways more serious, and concerns possible legal constraints if the protocols are not adhered to. Each of these problems can be overcome, and the whole process can be kept within the professional sphere — with one important proviso, that of the profession's demonstrating its ability to deal with doctors who do not perform to an adequate standard. This has been referred to already; but no apology is made for raising it again.

A further issue is relevant to both medical audit and its educational implications; and it picks up a theme described earlier, that of the ownership of the data. This is a particularly sensitive issue if in the process of audit particularly poor results are noted. If audit is performed and results are conveyed in a confidential manner, then there is the opportunity for the doctor whose performance is questioned to change and improve without public criticism's becoming necessary. Indeed the whole principle of postgraduate and continuing medical education is based on this. But what about the public? Are they not entitled to know if a particular doctor is not up to standard? What about management and the use of scarce resources? These questions are at the heart of the debate on CME, and relate to whether or not the profession can regulate its own activities, or whether an outside body is required — whether the medical profession can be trusted or not, and whether it can provide effective and efficient remedial action to those who require it. If the confidentiality of the data is lost, doctors may not co-operate. If there is no real improvement in performance, the public will have a right to be informed. Herein lies the importance of CME and the role of medical audit.

10.7   The role of the medical society in CME

Medical societies of all sorts occur throughout the world. They often began as dining societies, as debating societies, or even as ways of sharing a library. Many of them began at the end of the eighteenth century or the beginning of the nineteenth, and some are still functioning. They are of two main types, general or specialist. The general ones bring together a wide range of doctors, and tend to have a syllabus which will attract a wide audience, both general practitioners and consultants. They provide a general meeting-place for the exchange of views and for sharing experience. While the society usually has as its objective the increasing of knowledge amongst its members, it is often the informal social contact at the meeting rather than the formal presentation which is of the greatest value. Such societies thus fulfil one of the important functions described in the section on how doctors learn. The social function of these events should not be underestimated, as they provide an informal support mechanism for doctors, and allow for the sharing of information and problems.

The specialist societies provide a similar function, but have a more defined audience. They provide a way of rapidly exchanging information and of presenting new ideas to an informed and critical peer group. The audit function is therefore strong, and there is the ability to present results and to compare them with those of others. In recent years there has been an enormous expansion in the number of specialist societies, each becoming more specialist than the next. There are obviously clear advantages in this, as they bring together like-minded and committed individuals, who can provide a professional focus for the group. The disadvantages are also clear, in that links with other specialties are avoided, and general developments in medicine may be neglected. Every specialist has stories about other doctors who clearly are not up to date with their particular interest. It is for this reason that there needs to be a mechanism by which regular exchange of information can occur. Another challenge for CME.

10.8 Conclusions

1. This chapter has focused on some of the important issues which are currently relevant to CME. Looking ahead to the future raises other matters which have a bearing on broader educational issues. The first is one which has already been discussed: that of interprofessional

education. For many of the reasons noted above, this should be encouraged. There will need to be evidence of increased trust between professional groups; but the potential advantages are great. Somehow a mechanism must be found to facilitate this exchange of experience.

2. A second major issue must lie in the assessment of the effectiveness and efficiency of the educational process. There is a need for educational research which brings together the theoretical base and relates it, via practical programmes, to the outcome of patient care. Medical audit, or more properly clinical audit, is one powerful tool which might be more widely used.

3. A third major issue is to consider further the overall agenda for CME, and question whether it should be left to individual doctors to determine the 'curriculum', or whether there should be other input — for example, a role for the public in determining standards and the outcome of care. As an extension of this there may be a case for positively influencing the direction of education. Thus there could be a positive attempt to make doctors more interested in health rather than illness, or to ensure that all doctors had some education in the principles of management.

Such initiatives could have a profound effect on the way in which medicine is practised and on the outcome of patient care. The challenge to set that agenda is one for all those concerned with medical education.

Bibliography

Belsheim, D. J. (1986). Models for continuing professional education. *Medical Education*, **61**, 971–8.

Berwick, D. M. (1989). Continuous improvement as an ideal in health care. *New England Journal of Medicine*, **320**, 53–6.

Department of Health (1990). *The quality of medical care: report of the standing medical advisory committee*. HMSO, London.

Green, J. S., Grosswald, S. J., Suter, E., and Walthall, D. B. (ed.) (1984). *Continuing education for the health professions*. Jossey-Bass, London.

Greenfield, S. (1989). The state of outcome research: are we on target? *New England Journal of Medicine*, **320**, 1142–3.

Jarvis, P. (1983). *Professional education*. Croom Helm, London.

Kings Fund Centre (1990). *Medical audit — a hospital handbook*.

Linzer, M. (1987). The journal club and medical education. *Postgraduate Medical Journal*, **63**, 475–8.

Tarlov, A. R. (1989). The medical outcomes study. *Journal of the American Medical Association*, **262**, 925–30.

11 *The contribution of general practice*
James McCormick

Much has been written about the contribution of general practice to undergraduate education. This is not an attempt to rehearse yet again the detail, which can be accessed in some of the references at the end of the chapter.

It was once fashionable to write out educational objectives, and in some places it may still be so. These were usually divided into knowledge, skills, and attitudes, and were stated in the form 'the student shall be able to . . .'. For example, 'the student shall be able to describe the symptoms and causes of renal colic', 'the student shall be able to demonstrate the ability to hear and describe heart sounds', 'the student shall demonstrate a concern for patient's legitimate privacy'. In the end this often appeared a time-consuming and to some extent a futile exercise, even when it was supplemented by statements as to how these educational objectives were to be taught and assessed. These detailed objectives were often supplemented by broad aims or goals — so broad as to be little more than almost meaningless or tautologous aspirations.

None the less, education cannot be succesfully pursued unless there exists at least some notion of the end-product which is desired. As a general rule in universities it seems that the nature of the desired end-product need never be made explicit: it can be left to take care of itself. The present chapter is an attempt to steer a middle course between the mindless detail of some educational objectives and totally ignoring the problem of what that end-product might reasonably be.

It starts from the premiss that the growth of knowledge, much of which is trivial and evanescent rather than seminal and permanent, has distorted medical education. The distortion is the result of failure to appreciate that it is because available medical knowledge has far outstripped one man's comprehension that education becomes essential. When knowledge is sparse education may remain a luxury. A plumber can acquire the knowledge and skills to be effective without the luxury of education. An ill-educated medical profession daily demonstrates the abuse of knowledge which results from the denigration of judgement.

11.1 The role of the doctor

Roles are determined by the cultures and values of societies. For example, the role of father has undergone dramatic change in our society within a brief period of time. It is now expected that fathers will play a much more active part in the care of infants and small children, and fathers who reject this as part of their role may expect at least some degree of opprobrium.

By contrast with the role of father, the role of doctor has undergone relatively little change. Much of the role is a response to a universal need for individuals who are able to mediate between our illnesses and diseases and their consequences. Even the most primitive societies identify individuals, witch-doctors and shamans, who are invested with special powers and gifts. This is part of the universal need for explanations which is the *raison d'être* of religions. Religions exist to provide explanations for our birth, our death, and the nature of the journey in between. With the decline in orthodox religious belief doctors are now expected to provide such explanations, as well as to alleviate suffering, and, it sometimes seems, to postpone death indefinitely.

Both the real and the imagined benefits of the spectacular growth in scientific knowledge have created a climate, often fostered by doctors, of illusory faith in the power of modern medicine. Lewis Thomas has remarked that 'the ship of biological science is under way, but only just'. The educated doctor must recognize that the knowledge which he possesses, which is of a different order from that of his patients, largely defines his ignorance, and provides little justification for an inflated ego.

The role of doctor in our society is still invested with the expectation of personal care and a commitment which transcends that of most other professional relationships. This may be summarized as 'putting the patient first'. Society expects doctors to respond to emergencies, even at the expense of other prior social commitments. It expects surgeons to complete operations with all possible care, and to be oblivious of being late for dinner or late on the first tee.

Personal care includes expectations of undivided attention, of courtesy, and of being called by name (which should, however, preclude the unmandated use of Christian names so prevalent in the care of the elderly.) Included is the belief that the injunction of the Hippocratic Oath to keep secret information divulged in the consultation will be honoured.

Because society invests doctors with special powers it does not expect them to behave as other men. They are expected to be sober (except while they remain students), not to be foulmouthed, not to be discovered in adultery, and not to be primarily interested in making money.

The educated doctor, aware of the role which society imposes, will develop coping mechanisms to deal with the inevitable conflicts which the expectations of the patients will produce in his personal and professional life.

11.2 The aim of the doctor

Many doctors, very reasonably, have as their aim that they should make sufficient money, without excessive trauma, to keep them and their families in the state to which they feel entitled. That is the reason that they opted for medicine as a career. If this aim is paramount, or more important, is made overt, it is in conflict with the expectations of society. As a result this aim is little talked about in medical schools, and there is ambivalence towards those students who nakedly confess that they would as lief have been businessmen, but thought that the prospects in medicine were brighter.

If the aim of a farmer is to make a living by growing food, what does the doctor aspire to do in order to justify being paid? Since time immemorial these aspirations have included the treatment of disease and the alleviation of suffering. Because of the placebo effect, all treatments alleviate symptoms; but only recently have treatments which affect disease become available to the profession. Even when therapies were ineffective, and often harmful, at least some physicians were held in high regard. Therapeutic activism is still rampant, sometimes nowadays with great benefit to people, as in many surgical procedures and in the management of diabetes and thyroid disorders, for example — but often without clear indications. Both doctors and patients are unhappy with therapeutic inactivity, which is perceived as therapeutic nihilism.

More recently, the prevention of disease and the promotion of health have been added to the treatment of established disease and the alleviation of pain as a major aim of doctors. Much of this activity, particularly screening for cancers and risk-markers for coronary heart disease, is based on false premises, and has not fulfilled its promises. It has wasted resources and been the cause of iatrogenic harm. The idea of the promotion of health should surely prompt some question as to the nature of the health which is being promoted. As our longevity is, for the most part, encoded in our genes, and because we all suffer from that sexually transmitted disease which is life itself, ill-advised health promotion is a cause of holy dread and inappropriate anxiety, rather than a contribution to well-being.

The educated doctor must appreciate the true extent of his ignorance, and must be equipped to distinguish between the placebo effect and specific therapies and between reality and wishful thinking.

11.3   The skill role

Educationists make a distinction between knowledge and skills; but under this present heading knowledge can also conveniently be regarded as part of the equipment a doctor needs to fulfil his aims. As possession of all medical knowledge is an unachievable goal the educated doctor must recognize the limitations of his or her existing knowledge, and recognize those others who can make good the deficiency. People who are asked about what they require from their doctors always put competence first; and this is followed by 'knowing when to refer'. Much is made of the need for lifelong learning and keeping up to date. However, the educated doctor recognizes that much that is new is evanescent, and will distinguish between true advances and transient fashion. He or she will also recognize the need to be aware of what is both new and worth while in fields other than one's own.

There are, of course, many skills which are necessary and important, and which are emphasized in both undergraduate and postgraduate training. These extend from the — relatively neglected — skills of achieving rapport and listening so that the patient has the opportunity to 'tell you the diagnosis', to the manual dexterities required to examine the nervous system or to undertake coronary artery surgery.

Educated doctors are needed because only the educated can aspire to full professional development. Professional development is a phrase which describes the possibility that training and experience, instead of ensuring that the same mistakes are made with increasing confidence, will allow continuing growth, maturity, wisdom, and judgement. J. K. Galbraith remarked that 'the denigration of value judgement is one of the mechanisms by which the scientific establishment maintains its misconceptions'. (The addition of value to judgement is an unfortunate tautology which has done the importance of judgement a great disservice.) Because individual people are unique, complex, and full of fears both rational and irrational (as seen by others), advising them in relation to matters which affect their health requires, as well as knowledge and skills, judgement — judgement which balances possible harms against possible benefits, and which recognizes that diseased or unhappy people are more than disordered machinery. The growth of knowledge has displaced judgement and threatened medical education. Unless education is revived at the expense of training, future generations of doctors will continue to harm their patients not from ignorance, but from stupidity.

11.4   The contribution of general practice

A popular definition of general practice begins with the statement that a general practitioner is a physician who provides 'personal, primary, and continuing care'. The unique contribution of general practice to the education of doctors relates to these tasks.

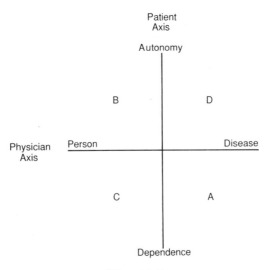

Fig. 11.1

11.5 Personal care

Most people in the National Health Service who are referred to hospital do not recognize a contract with an individual specialist, although his or her name may appear on the cover of their case-notes. They speak of 'attending the hospital', 'going to Accident and Emergency', 'being in St Whatever's', not of seeing Mr X or Dr Y. (One of the main reasons for the survival of private practice is that this allows a contract with a named individual and some measure of control.)

By contrast, most people who speak of 'my doctor' are referring to a general practitioner, and not only will be familiar with his or her name, but will expect that they shall be recognized by name, and by much else, by their familiar physician. This remains largely true despite the growth of group practices and the use of deputizing services.

The hospital is primarily concerned with diseases and their diagnosis and treatment: general practice is primarily concerned with people and their problems, which may include their diseases.

Figure 11.1 has two axes, a person axis which runs from autonomy to dependence, and a physician axis which runs from person-oriented to disease-oriented. Most of clinical medical education takes place in quadrant A, in which the physician is more concerned with diseases than with people, and in which patients have sacrificed, sometimes willingly and wisely, their autonomy, and are almost entirely dependent. (If I have to undergo cardiac surgery I do not want discussions about best procedures: I must become as a child and invest my trust in the surgeon, who should be God or God's first cousin, otherwise I would be mad to let him do it.)

On the other hand, for those suffering from a chronic or incurable condition, or those close to death, health is only possible if they are treated in quadrant B. Their right to autonomy includes the right to information (a right they may voluntarily relinquish), a right to decline treatment, and a right to 'call the shots'.

There is a danger that general practitioners treat patients, particularly the elderly, within quadrant C. This has many similarities between the relationship between parent and child, and is often tinged with mutual love.

Patients, usually from the United States, occasionally occupy Quadrant D. As a general rule doctors in these islands resent being treated as servants. This position is related to status and the payment of fees, both of which enhance patient control.

Those trained exclusively in hospitals, with their partly legitimate preoccupation with working in quadrant A, tend to be relatively unaware of the psychological component of having, or imagining oneself having, a disease. Those experienced in general practice recognize that the commonest reason for a consultation is reassurance about the meaning of symptoms. They are also aware of people's need to remain 'sick', that is to take up the 'sick role', and thus become entitled to escape their social obligations.

As part of their assessment our students are obliged to write an essay which stems from their undergraduate attachment to general practice. They almost without exception, comment upon the different relationship which exists between doctor and patient in general practice when compared with that which they have observed in hospital. This might be summed up in a note I received from one of our brightest students at the end of his time with us: he wrote 'thank you for showing me the human face of medicine'.

General practitioners suffer from a delusion that they have exclusive possession of 'the milk of human kindness'; this is of course nonsense, and many consultants are better than their general practitioner colleagues in recognizing the needs of people as people, as well as in dealing with their diseases. None the less, the tales that patients bring back from hospital, the day-to-day experience of students, the nature of hospital staffing, with many juniors being directly involved with patient care, provide ample and reliable evidence that personal doctoring is the exception rather than the rule.

Personal doctoring is about recognizing the unique nature of personal identity, and such recognition is an essential background to proper responses to anxiety, information-giving, and co-operation in treatment. As a result academic departments of general practice tend to emphasize what are known in the jargon of the moment as 'communication skills'. Probably more important is the 'hidden curriculum', which as Marshall Marinker pointed out, is unconsciously taught by the way doctors behave, by what they do 'not only on their lips but in their lives'. Personal care implies a relationship between patient and doctor at a level which transcends technical competence in the sense of skilful plumbing. Its advantages derive from improved communication and mutual knowledge and trust; its disadvantages from the creation of mutual dependence. Not only are patients dependent on their doctors, but doctors on their patients. In fee-paying societies they depend on patients for their income; in all societies they depend on patients for the maintenance of their self-esteem.

Within hospital it sometimes seems that the aspiration of most juniors is to meet the requirements of their seniors rather than the requirements of their patients. The good regard of their chiefs is more important to career advancement than the good regard of the patients whom they serve.

Lectures are a poor way of demonstrating the importance and value of personal care: it must be taught for the most part by means of observation which is subsequently reinforced by reflection — reflection which good teachers should encourage by providing a format in which it can take place. General practice can demonstrate to all potential doctors the value of personal care.

11.6 Primary care

Primary care is defined for my purposes as those aspects of health care services which are directly accessible to the public. Within the National Health Service only the Accident and Emergency departments of hospitals offer primary care; otherwise, access to hospital is by referral. General practitioners are not the only primary care providers: dentists, friendly neighbourhood pharmacists, nurses, and health visitors also provide primary care; none the less, general practitioners are the most significant doctors who offer care at the patient's discretion.

The reasons that people decide to consult doctors may be listed as: reassurance, diagnosis, treatment, the legitimization of the sick-role, 'problems of living with the human condition', the prevention of disease, and the surveillance of chronic conditions. The population of patients which is referred to hospital is a subset of that which attends general practitioners, a subset in which serious disease is overrepresented and people's other needs underrepresented. As a result, medical students whose clinical experience is confined to hospital, often in highly specialized units, have a distorted view of the prevalence of disease in the community and of people's real needs. This brings in its wake errors in diagnosis and the inappropriate use of investigations. Diagnosis depends to a large extent on prior probability, and tests only become reliable discriminators when the prevalence of target disorders lies between 20 and 80 per cent. It also leads to neglect of people's need for reassurance, of the importance of sick-role behaviour, and of the fact that not everyone who seeks professional help has a disease, as distinct from dis-ease.

Only experience in general practice can aspire to correct these important, and if all a doctor's experience has been in hospital, potentially permanent distortions of reality.

11.7 Continuing care

Despite increasing mobility within our society, many people have a relationship with their practitioner which extends over years. This relationship is rarely continuous, but more often episodic. None the less, the accumulation of episodes leads to the development of a relationship in which mutual knowledge has the chance to develop and in which the patient's past experience provides a basis for trust. 'Last time he said that I would get better and I did.' Such continuing care can encompass many of life's major events: birth, death, bereavement, marriage, and divorce. Such sharing, if only at some superficial level, creates a special relationship. Such relationships are by no means universal, but are sufficiently important that all doctors need to be aware of them, and of their strengths and weaknesses.

11.8 Teaching clinical skills

It has become apparent to many that the teaching hospital has become an environment which is inimical to the acquisition of the core clinical skills of history taking and physical examination. Patients are admitted for very short periods of time and many of them are acutely ill. The growth of day surgery and day hospitals will aggravate this situation even further. As a consequence there is much talk, and a little action, about transferring this central part of a medical student's experience from the hospital to the setting of general practice. Despite, generally unreasonable, fears about general practitioner's competence to do such teaching and reasonable fears within academic general practice about adequate resources to meet the challenge, there is every probability that this movement will grow and in time become the norm.

11.9 Teaching general practice

General practice as a specialty should be learned as a postgraduate and there is no place for attempting to teach general practice to undergraduates. Yet the temptation to do so is strong and aggravated by the reluctance of other disciplines to make a distinction between what is relevant to undergraduates and attempting to create embryo specialists. The idea of the safe general practitioner at graduation has been replaced by the idea of the safe intern but the notion of the omnicompetent, as distinct from the omnipotent, graduate is only dying by slow degrees.

11.10 The future

It is difficult to escape the conclusion that in the future general practice will have a much enhanced role in undergraduate education, both as a discipline and as an environment for education. Unfortunately most academic departments are small and underresourced, and at a time of economic recession additional resource can only come from redeployment, which is neither popular or easy. Furthermore, because of their emphasis on teaching, which on the whole has been much more imaginative than the approaches of their colleagues in other disciplines, and relies heavily on a small group format, research has taken second place. In a school that measures success by published papers in refereed journals small departments of general practice inevitably compare poorly with some other departments. However, failure to recognize the importance of general practice to undergraduate medical education will result in a perpetuation of an inherently unsatisfactory situation.

11.11 Conclusions

These noble sentiments make little contribution to problem-solving. Medical education is in a mess, and if the sentiments are to lead to improvement radical change is required — radical change which might be achievable by evolution rather than revolution. The essential requirement is a reduction in the content of basic medical education — a reduction which carries as a corollary earlier specialist training. Three or four years should suffice to educate an omnicompetent doctor, who would then enter specialist training in a chosen field, surgery, internal medicine, general practice, radiology, pathology, or whatever. In effect a general practitioner will not be expected to spend inadequate periods of time in specialist departments acquiring a useless degree of knowledge of pathology, microbiology, eye disease, or obstetrics. Instead the aspiring general practitioner would receive appropriate training in common eye diseases, common skin diseases, and the appropriate use of antibiotics in primary care. The aspiring specialist in internal medicine would not be obliged to spend time learning rudimentary antenatal care or orthopaedics, and the aspiring specialist in histopathology would not spend time flirting with psychology, the clinical care of children, or the management of mental illness.

It will be obvious that this is a variation, extension, or restatement of the idea of a core curriculum. It involves much earlier career choices; and it is therefore important that provision is made for change of career at some later stage. A core curriculum, designed to educate rather than to train, would be very different from that inflicted upon present-day undergraduates.

Bibliography

Skrabanek, P. and McCormick, J. (1989). *Follies and fallacies in medicine*. Tarragon Press, Glasgow.

Association of University Teachers of General Practice. (1984). Undergraduate medical education in general practice, Occasional paper 28. Royal College of General Practitioners, London.

Fraser, R. C. (1991). Undergraduate medical education: present state and future needs. *British Medical Journal*, **303**, 41–3.

Part III: Challenges

12 *Consumers and patients*

12.1 Some cases

12.1.1

Dr G has been qualified for many years, and is well liked by all. One of his female patients in her twenties has a problem which has not been responding well to treatment. She approaches him saying that she has read in a magazine about some new tablets for her condition. Dr G feels rather irritated, partly because he has not himself heard of the treatment, and partly because he feels that patients have no right to suggest their own medicine. He wonders what to do, and tells her that he has had fifteen years' experience and knows what is best for her.

12.1.2

Dr H comes from a medical family. His father had been a dedicated GP and his mother had been a nurse and eventually his father's receptionist. His uncle, now retired, had been a surgeon. There was never any question but that Dr H would become a doctor, and he has just passed through medical school and is in training as a GP. He was very upset to find that some meetings of the partnership were concerned with how to get rid of elderly patients who were likely to become expensive and a drain on the practice budget, and how to take on young and healthy patients. When he questioned these policies he was told: 'You've got to enter the real world — we're all businessmen now.'

12.2 Doctors' duties and patients' rights

These cases really contain two challenges to medical education, which are connected but separable. The first is the challenge from patient autonomy, or the desire of patients to have more information and in general to be more involved in decisions on their treatment; the second is the challenge from the market-place, or the need for medicine to be a cost-effective service, with all that that entails. Both challenges are being encouraged by the British Government, and both can be discussed under the heading of 'consumerism'; but there are important differences between the two challenges, and the second is a much more serious challenge than the first. The first represents a challenge to those traditional medical *attitudes* that students unconsciously assimilate at medical schools. We have discussed this process of assimilation of traditional values in Chapter 4. But the second represents a challenge to the *financial infrastructure* of medicine, and the change in attitudes which it is likely to bring about in both doctors and patients is likely to be more violent and more radical. Let us look first at what we have called the challenge from patient autonomy.

The traditional attitude of medicine (which we have already discussed in Chapter 3) contains a central element which might be expressed as follows:

● *The overriding obligation of the doctor is to treat her/his own patients to the best of her/his ability.*

In other words, doctors have traditionally seen themselves as dedicated professionals providing a round-the clock service to their patients — but that service is conceived in terms of the medical perception of patients' needs.

The traditional attitude can survive several important modifications. For example, the idea of good treatment can be enlarged to include improved doctor–patient communication. Again, the individualistic, possessive ring of 'his/her own patients' can be changed into a more harmonious chime by introducing the idea of teams. The treatment of patients can be and is increasingly being shared by teams. It is true that many doctors express irritation at being lumped together with others as 'health professionals'; but there is no question that increasingly health care is being delivered by teams. None the less, the teams are led by doctors, and the crucial decisions are made by doctors. In other words, we have a modification rather than a change in the traditional attitude.

The same conclusion can be reached if we stress the role of the doctor in providing preventive services or in health education. These developments involve the enlargement, but not the radical alteration, of the traditional attitude of beneficence, which is respected by a large number of patients.

This attitude, however, has also been challenged over the past twenty years, and the challenge can be expressed as follows: *The provision of health-care is pre-eminently a matter of patients' rights to medical services, and doctors' duties should reflect this.* The main idea behind this approach is that of personal autonomy. It should be assumed, according to this approach, that patients, like anyone else, are self-determining, self-governing people who are able to make up their own minds on appropriate treatment for themselves, provided doctors supply enough information. Emphasis in this approach is on the informed consent of the patient to any treatment offered.

If we were looking in detail at this approach it would be necessary to devote a large amount of discussion to questions such as the standard of information disclosure which is appropriate. Is it, for example, what patients happen in variable ways to want? Is it the standard of disclosure which would be typical of professional peers? Is it what the abstract 'reasonable person' might want? Similar questions can be raised about the nature of the voluntariness involved in informed consent. And there are obviously difficult questions about the elderly, the mentally handicapped, young children, and so on. These and many other questions related to the full articulation of the new attitude have been discussed by others. Our question is not here one of detailed analysis of the new attitude but of main principle. Can the traditional attitude which has been, and to some extent still is, communicated by medical education be modified by this new approach without radical distortion?

Our view is that it can. Indeed, the need for a changed approach is already being met, for many medical schools now require courses which discuss such matters as patient access to medical records, communication skills, breaking bad news, and so on. We have advocated an increased attention to this aspect of medical education, and have also suggested that this 'whole-person' approach can be improved by the inclusion or encouragement of the humanities in medical education.

We can sum this up if we say that the first element in the challenge to medical education from consumerism consists of a stress on the rights, or the autonomy, of patients. But we hold that this challenge can be met without a radical change in the traditional 'ethos' of medicine that we have discussed in Chapter 4. The challenge can be met if medical education stresses partnership rather than paternalism. This change can be assimilated into medical practice because patients remain patients, except that they have heightened awareness of their rights as consumers of health care, and doctors are able to take cognizance of this.

12.3 Medical practice as a business

In terms of the second and more radical challenge to medical education from the position of consumerism the financial considerations of being a consumer come into the foreground; and equally the financial implications of the doctor as a supplier of medical services come into the foreground. This is a radical challenge, because traditionally doctors saw themselves as being, first and foremost, members of a profession; but now they are being encouraged by the Government to see themselves as businessmen. Patients are to become customers and doctors suppliers. In discussing this important development we must consider whether the changes are simply in terminology. Are the changes simply in political rhetoric, or are they likely to be in the substance which underlies medical education? What's in a name?

There are two approaches to the question of 'What's in a name?' which do not lead anywhere of interest; but since it is tempting to go down these roads, it may be helpful to show why each is a cul-de-sac.

12.3.1 *The definitional approach*

It is not uncommon to assume that it is possible to determine what something is by using a dictionary. Thus a dictionary may tell us that a patient means (among other things) someone who goes to a medical practitioner, and a customer or consumer is someone who goes to a retailer. It seems to follow that these are two different concepts with nothing in common; and indeed the same might be thought to follow even if we adopt more sophisticated sociological definitions of each. But it is not possible to stop social and economic change by using a dictionary. The important question is rather whether patients are nowadays adopting some of the characteristics of consumers, and whether they should be encouraged to do so. Equally, we can ask whether doctors should be encouraged to see themselves as suppliers of services in a market.

Before we leave the unfruitful question of definitions we should also note a danger of the new rhetoric of health care — that the term 'consumer' becomes like the abstraction of the economic textbook 'rational economic man'. The truth is that consumers come in all shapes and sizes, and can be disabled, mentally handicapped, elderly, etc. In other words, we are not comparing just two concepts — the patient and the consumer — but a host of related concepts. So while it might be possible for *some* patients to adopt the characteristics of some consumers, it may not be possible for other patients to be like any consumer.

12.3.2   The moral high ground

The professions generally, and the medical profession in particular, sometimes approach the idea of business from a position of moral superiority. This superiority can be articulated in detail through a series of contrasts:

The professions	Businessmen (the 'market')
The professions promote the interests of patients, clients, etc.	Businessmen promote their own interests, not those of customers.
Fees are incidental to professional activity.	Profits are central to business activity.
The professions are concerned with real 'needs' of the public or important aspects of human life, such as 'health', 'justice', or 'education'.	Business is concerned with wants or preferences (often trivial).
The professions have a duty to comment on broad matters of public policy.	Business has no such public or social function.
The professions have a political and commercial independence which makes their comments relevant to public policy.	Business lacks independence, and its comments on public policy express vested interests or right-wing politics.
The professions have a knowledge-base which requires a broad education.	Business has a shallower, opportunistic knowledge-base, for which 'training' is a more appropriate term than education.

These contrasts create a sense of moral superiority in the professions, to which businessmen respond aggressively with claims such as 'We live in the real world, not in a ivory tower', or 'We earn the wealth of the country on which the professions depend', or 'At least we are honest about the need to make a profit.' But the validity of the contrasts can be questioned: some are based on conceptual confusions, and others are outdated by changes in the knowledge-base of business and a changed economic structure in society.

Take first the issues of self-interest and profits. The idea here is that, on the one hand, the patient is vulnerable in that he/she lacks information and may be sick, so that the doctor is able to provide a service to the patient within a framework of professionalized beneficence; whereas, on the other hand, the trader and the consumer are on an equal footing and can then, directly or indirectly, establish the best deal which suits the balance of their respective self-interests. But, to be fair, the contrasts must be drawn at the same points in the chain of service. The professional is described as beneficent at the point where the service is delivered — during actual patient-care. But this is compatible with saying that professional contracts for services rendered are actually being negotiated at another point in the chain in a self-interested manner. Equally, a business will establish its prices in a self-interested way — the astute businessman will consider what price the market will stand; but that is compatible with saying that at the point of delivery of service a salesman may offer impartial advice on what would best suit the requirements of the customer.

It is simply a muddle to contrast the benign service at which the doctor aims with the self-interested profit at which the businessman aims. The doctor supplies medical services in a benign way; but doctors are also fee-earners, and it would be disingenuous to pretend that their professional associations do not attempt to maximize their fees. Equally, businessmen are also suppliers of the goods and services necessary for the well-being of social life, and it is unfair to suggest that at the point of delivery there is no attempt to provide a service fitting the needs of the consumer.

Consider, secondly, the contrast between the alleged ideals served by the professions and the 'trifles of frivolous utility' offered by the market. Sometimes this contrast is stated as one between important human *needs* — health, justice, or education — and superficial human *wants* or *preferences*. But this is unfair too. There are trivial sides to the professions — the cosmetics of health care or the frivolities of litigation; whereas the market characteristically supplies the necessities without which we cannot exist, and generates the wealth on which we all depend.

A third difference sometimes stressed between business and the professions concerns the alleged social function of the professions. It is clear that the health professions will be concerned with the interests of *specific* patients; but they also have a broader social function. For example, doctors have a duty to speak out on broad issues of health, as for example they might speak out against cigarette advertising.

But businessmen too can have a wider social function outside the concerns of their specific industries. Bodies such as the Confederation of British Industry are widely recognized as having the function of commenting on broad matters of social utility; and industry is increasingly involved in such matters as the sponsorship of the arts.

Fourthly, take the matter of independence. There was an historical period when it might have been claimed that only the professions had the political and commercial independence which enabled their comments to be disinterested. But this is no longer true. All the professions are in varying ways dependent on both governments and/or commercial support. For example, the medical profession is obviously dependent on the Government for its major funding. Moreover, there is a suspicion that drug companies also control at least some of the activities of the medical profession. On the other hand, whereas the primary duty of individual companies is to their shareholders, and national bodies such as the CBI are clearly commercial pressure groups, they can still speak their mind on broad policy issues, and are not necessarily more subservient to the Government than the British Medical Association.

Finally, it is certainly important that members of the professions should be educated as distinct from merely trained men and women. But the professions no longer have a monopoly of educated men and women. Large numbers of graduates enter industry, business, and finance; and indeed if we consider the complexities of decision-making involved at all levels it is clear that management of all sorts requires educated as well as trained men and women.

The conclusion of this section is that the traditional contrast between the professions and business is based on a misunderstanding of the present position of each group. As we move into the next century it is plain that there is going to be much more overlap, and that the professions have much to learn from business. It is therefore important to clear away uninformed, confused, or emotionally-based prejudice. It is also important to consider just what and how much the medical profession can learn from business, and that will be the concern of the next section of this chapter.

12.4   What can the medical profession learn from business?

The Government, in a White Paper entitled *Working for patients*, is encouraging the medical profession to see their profession as a business. The hope is that there will be conspicuous improvements from the establishment of an internal market in health-care services. What are these hoped-for improvements, and are there signs that they are likely to be achieved as the decade progresses towards the year 2000? There are three connected aspects of medical care where we might expect to see improvements with the establishment of an internal market: patient choice; quality of service; and expenditure.

If patients are to be encouraged to see themselves as consumers or as customers then one obvious benefit which should be expected is improved choice. One criticism of medical services of all kinds, which has grown in volume from the 1970s on, is that they are essentially paternalistic. To be paternalistic is to decide for others what they have a right to decide for themselves. Medical paternalism is thought to exist at two levels: at the point of delivery of the service (in the doctor–patient) relationship), and in the selection of priorities in what is to be delivered (whether emphasis in the provision of services is to be, for example, on acute services or on the care of the elderly or of the mentally handicapped). Will the much-vaunted internal market improve patients' choice in either of these respects?

There seems little sign that this is happening. In the first type of situation — the doctor–patient relationship — choice *cannot* be achieved by a market mechanism, but only by the education of the doctor and the patient through improved communication. The greater the patient's information the more meaningful the choice, and the closer the doctor and the patient come to equality. This improvement can come about only through changes in medical education, and indeed through the education of patients (for it is certainly the case that many patients prefer that their doctor should choose for them). It is not at all clear how such a change could come about through the introduction of a market mechanism. Without information choice is empty, and the poor and the disadvantaged in particular require to be informed to enable choice to be meaningful. Markets cannot help here.

When we move to the question of priorities in the provision of services, however, it is possible that market mechanisms can do more to improve choice. They can do so if patients, or at least bodies such as local health councils, patients' groups, etc., are allowed to participate in decision-making in the establishment of these priorities. For example, do we, the consumers, want a heart-transplant unit or do we want improved services for the mentally handicapped? The answer at present is that we have no choice. Decisions are made for political reasons, or as the result of powerful medical lobbies; they are not made by consumers. But local health councils could do a lot here. It is worth noting that *Working for patients* speaks of giving patients greater choice among the services that are available. But we might also want greater choice in *what* services are made available. (It might of course be argued that this is a *citizenship* rather than a *consumer* issue. The point is a nice one, but the issue remains.)

Where, then, is patient choice thought to exist? Patients can choose what breakfast cereal they want in hospital! More seriously, they can choose their GP. But the latter choice can cut both ways. GPs with an eye to their budgets will not be anxious to accept high-cost patients such as the elderly. It is not likely that one should be able to change patients into consumers without also changing their GPs into consumers.

Moreover, there is a serious risk of creating what economists call 'supply-induced demand'. To the extent that GP fees are linked to the supply of certain services, such as screening programmes, there is a danger that people will be encouraged to think that participation in these programmes is essential for their health, when in reality it is essential for GP fees. There are examples of this in the USA. In short, in terms of any possible increase in patients' choice the introduction of business terminology has achieved little.

In the second place, is the introduction of an internal market likely to improve the quality of medical services? Answers to this question will vary in accordance with the nature of those who are monitoring the services. In many of the large public services, such as British Telecom, the Post Office, or British Gas, there are consumer councils which monitor service. Those bodies have many lay members. In smaller businesses quality control is provided by the discipline of the market — competition from rivals. What happens in medical services? How are standards of care monitored? The position of the British Government is that 'the quality of medical work can be reviewed only by a doctor's peers' (*Working paper on medical audit*). This does not sound like consumerism gone mad! It sounds more like the expression of a paternalistic monopoly. And what is being measured? Medical audit tends to stress outcomes; but what comes out depends very much on what goes in. The most important input is the quality of service in treatment. It is much harder to establish quality assurance here. Moreover, the whole issue of outcomes and quality of care is especially difficult in areas such as terminal care or antenatal care. The users of medical services, or their relatives or representatives, require to be empowered not only in the choice of the services they wish to use, but also in the matter of evaluating the quality of those services.

The third area which was expected to improve through the introduction of a market is expenditure. Will a business approach to medicine cut costs as the decade progresses towards the year 2000?

In answering this question we must avoid an oversimplification. It is easy to have a simple version of the market relationship in which we are thinking of two parties only — the trader and the customer. But traders obtain their goods from whole-salers and manufacturers, and the market relationship holds there as well. In health care the market is one between differ-ent sets of managers — the managers of purchasing health authorities and the managers of provider units. The taxpayer may benefit here from cost-cutting — a reasonable objective; but the direct benefits to the patients or the users could only be marginal if we consider the increased cost of administration.

Some conclusions have emerged from this section of the paper. First, both the professions and business are evolving in this last decade of the century; and, in particular, concepts from business, such as information, choice, quality control, and cost-cutting can be used to improve medical services. There is a danger, however, that these changes will not in all cases benefit patients. It is not, as some critics suggest, that the changes are cosmetic, or just political rhetoric; they are changes of sub-stance. The danger is more that we shall have a manager-driven consumerism rather than a patient-driven consumerism; and it is far from clear that the result will be a user-friendly service. If we are to have paternalism it may be preferable to have that of the old medical superintendent and GP to that of the general manager. A genuinely market-based medical service might free us from most sorts of paternalism; but the service must be modelled on the right areas of the market, or we shall simply be substituting managerial bureaucracy for medical paternalism.

12.5 The challenge to medical education

If these changes come about in the financial infrastructure of medicine they will certainly bring about changes in medical decision-making. Our question is the challenge they offer to medical education. The danger is that medical education will not change, and will continue to exude the traditional ethos. A serious gulf will then develop between how doctors see them-selves and how they actually behave in medical practice. We noted, however, that even if medicine is encouraged to adopt some of the practices and attitudes of business it can still hold a responsible attitude towards patients. As we tried to show, the difference between the professions and business cannot plausibly be described as the difference between a beneficent and a self-interested point of view. The truth may be that the traditional differences between the two are nowadays beginning to disappear, as each absorbs the good points of the other. The fact remains, however, that medicine must still treat the elderly, the mentally handicapped, and the chronically and the terminally ill. The absorption of business attitudes into medical education must not be allowed to obscure the central importance of patients who will make a loss in business terms. Nobody makes profits merely from the chronically sick; yet care for these patients is arguably a major concern for modern medicine.

There is another respect in which medicine should resist the ideals of business. Business by its very nature tends to expand. There are close connections between growth and profitability. Should medicine expand?

Here it is important to draw again the distinction we have already discussed (Chapter 3) between health *care* and *health*. The encouragement of consumerism is naturally concentrated on the provision and quality of health care; but the health of the nation is affected only marginally by health care. Health care can, perhaps, be seen in economic terms, as a commodity which can be handed from the top down in a paternalistic way, or bought across the counter in a consumer-orientated way. But health itself is in no sense a commodity, and cannot be acquired or enhanced in this way. There is an assumption in Government circles that if screening and preventive services are increased there will be an improvement in health. It is very doubtful, however, whether this will result. Improvements in health are more likely to come about through curbs on the sugar, alcohol, tobacco, and 'road' lobbies; and there is no sign that the Government is likely to tackle these. The evidence from the USA suggests that the more direct the link between the supply of medical services (including prevention and screening) and the payment of fees, the greater will be the spread and use of such services, and therefore the more people will come to see health in medical terms. One important message which medical education should convey to its students is that medical services can improve the health of only a fraction of the population. We stressed that the intrinsic aim of medicine is a narrow one; wider aims, such as reducing obesity, do not seem to be in general terms aims of *medicine*, but should be left to individuals to decide for themselves, assisted perhaps by non-medical educational services.

12.6 Conclusions

1. The concept of consumerism conceals two linked ideas: that of the informed patient in partnership with his/her doctor choosing appropriate treatment; and that of the customer or user of medical services which have cost implications.

2. Medical education can assimilate the change involved in incorporating the first of these ideas, and can encourage doctors who see patients as partners.

3. The second idea is more of an unknown, and seems to have far-reaching implications for the practice of medicine, and, therefore, for medical education. There is a danger that this fundamental change will completely alter the nature of the doctor–patient relationship; the changes cut both ways, and doctors are more powerful than patients.

4. It is important to stress, however, that business relationships can display many of the traditional characteristics of professional relationships, and that medical education has some lessons which it can learn from business practice.

5. The move to business practice in medicine must not be allowed to obscure the fact that health remains the responsibility of individuals, and must not be medicalized by the inappropriate spread of medical services.

Bibliography

Working for patients (1989). London, HMSO.
Working paper on medical audit (1989). London, HMSO.

13 Clinical freedom and a mind of one's own

13.1 A pharmaceutical nightmare

One day a dispensary student had been left to mind the store, and was confronted unexpectedly by a customer asking for a convenient remedy for aching feet. Anxious to approach the problem systematically rather than just handing over any old type of ointment, the student retired to the back room and looked up 'Feet (sore)' in the still-pristine volumes of his *Theory and practice for pharmacy students*. Here he discovered that the condition could seemingly be caused (although the authors are cautious in their use of that word) by anything from tightly fitting shoes to intermittent claudication. Disconcertingly, his book offered little guidance as to 'most likely explanations'. New suggestions about how to approach such problems had been slotted in alongside the old (some of the latter undoubtedly dating back to the alchemists), and no remedy had ever really gone out of date, or could be said to have been 'replaced' with something more effective. More worryingly, each of the aetiological accounts presented seemed logically to rule out all the others; but then this seemed to worry none of the contributors — least of all the editors.

Not understanding how he was expected to make use of such a guide, our student sought the author's preface. Here he was confronted with the view that given the 'uniqueness' of each of the conditions reported on, the ultimate choice had to be left to the individual dispenser: 'it all depends what works for you' ran the relevant paragraph.

Closing the book, and filled with a new enthusiasm, he reflected momentarily on his previous misconception. They were right, of course; he should have realized where his appetite for practical prescription was leading him; to theoretical synthesis, comparative evaluation of concepts, cumulative collections of theory, and the like. Mechanistic impositions on the freedom and creativity of the man at the practice interface. Much better to guess — flexibly and intuitively of course. He remembered from his lectures on Non-Directive Pharmacy the dangers attaching to the indiscriminate use of 'narrow empirical products', Jehu's Jelly, Skinner's Salve, and such. No, he must not seek to avoid his professional responsibilities: the choice was his alone, However, on returning to his shelves to look intuitively for likely remedies, he was faced with another setback. From the accompanying literature he discerned that most of the available mixtures had never been tested at all. Those which had were far from spectacular successes, he recalled, and had only been kept on the market for the sake of a few addicts. Just then our hovering student's attention was caught by a large volume sitting on the topmost shelf. It was entitled *Feet and Society*. A quick translation from it revealed that sore feet result from interaction with Pedestrian Transportation Facilities (pavements, as they are sometimes called by the non-technical). Furthermore, structural factors in late capitalist society determine that profit-motivated footwear suppliers are forced increasingly to skimp on their products at the expense of the oppressed consumer.

The student dashed from his dispensary eager to raise the consciousness of his customer with this new knowledge, but alas, she had tired of waiting and hobbled away (Sheldon 1978).

13.2 Clinical freedom

The desire to express individuality through professional judgement is expressed in the concept of 'clinical freedom'. This is a freedom which doctors have jealously guarded. How is it to be analysed, and how far is it worth cherishing? In answering this question we are examining another challenge to medical education, because clinical freedom is central to the ethos of medicine, and is part of the hidden agenda of medical education.

What is clinical freedom? We might suggest the following definition:

• *Clinical freedom is the freedom of a doctor to investigate, prescribe, or carry out a procedure, refer, or communicate, regardless of cost, other professional opinion, or patients', or social views, in the best interests of the patient.*

It can be seen that this is simply a slightly longer version of what was previously enunciated (12.2) as an articulation of the traditional medical attitude. Before we discuss it we shall refine our conceptual tools.

A distinction can be drawn between 'negative freedom' (freedom from external interference to do what you want) and 'positive freedom' (being enabled to do what you want). For example, a person might be free to enter a university, in the sense that there is no sort of prohibition on this, but lack the means to be able to do so, and in this sense not be free to do so.

Returning now to clinical freedom, we can note a number of negative constraints on clinical freedom. As we have seen in the last chapter, the requirement to inform patients of their diagnosis and proposed treatment and in general to involve them in partnership in their own treatment involves a constraint on the unfettered clinical freedom of the doctor. Secondly, cost is clearly becoming an increasingly large constraint on the clinical freedom of the doctor. Thirdly, the pressure of professional peers and the rest of the team are constraints. Fourthly, as medical law is developed it has become a constraint, and relatedly the influence of medical ethics has increased over the last decade. We have already discussed many of these factors, and list them again in this context to indicate the constraints on clinical freedom.

Let us turn now to positive freedom, or being enabled to exercise clinical judgement. This again depends on various factors. Most obviously it will depend on the negative factors in reverse. Thus the doctor is enabled to exercise clinical freedom if he has the resources and the patient's consent, and is supported by the team; if there is nothing legally or ethically wrong; and if he has the time. More interestingly, positive freedom is enhanced by knowledge and skills. Thus, a doctor is not free to make a certain clinical judgement or to carry out a certain procedure, or even to make a certain kind of referral, if he does not know of the existence of the procedure or cannot carry it out. In other words, knowledge increases (positive) clinical freedom. This generates an interesting paradox — that of being forced to be free (an idea deriving from Rousseau). There is a case for requiring doctors to attend in-service courses (thus infringing their negative freedom) in order to enrich their clinical judgement and so enhance their (positive) freedom. We have already discussed continuing and specialist medical education.

There is another aspect of clinical freedom in the positive sense. This aspect concerns the question of what the doctor is free to do *qua* doctor or *qua* clinician. For example, suppose a doctor were to say 'I think your unhappy marriage is the main factor in bringing about your illness. I advise you to leave your wife.' Is this different from the case of the bank manager who says 'I think your wife is the main factor bringing about your unhealthy bank balance. You should leave her'? Is it just that health is more important than a bank balance? Or a bank manager less important than a doctor? This raises the issue we have already discussed concerning the role of the doctor. It would be easy to think that the role of the doctor is wide or narrow according to the knowledge-base of medicine. This is false. The role of the doctor is largely determined by public expectations. Thus a nineteenth-century doctor might have a wide role, but narrow knowledge-base. We have argued for a narrow role in Chapter 3.

What is the value of clinical freedom? Note that we are not asking why doctors often defend it. This second question invites special pleading for the maintenance of outmoded ways of doing things and the protection of vested interests! We are asking what if anything is *valuable* about clinical freedom.

First, it might be suggested that clinical freedom is worth while for the same reason that any kind of freedom is — like autonomy, clinical freedom is worth while for its own sake. But it is very doubtful if *clinical* freedom is a good in itself. Yet surely it must be good, secondly, for what it *brings*, allegedly some service to patients not otherwise possible. Is it then an instrumental or enabling good (as distinct from an intrinsic good)? What does it bring to the clinical situation? Perhaps two main things. One related to the negative sense of freedom, and the other to the positive sense.

Let us take first clinical freedom in the negative sense. An emphasis on clinical freedom transfers the onus of justification to the party who would try to interfere with the doctor. It is not that clinical freedom is always a trump card (although many doctors clearly think it is); but that, for example, it is up to the government, or the law, or public opinion, or a given individual patient to show why doctors should not prescribe or act as they think appropriate. Often these public debates are good for doctors, for they force them to consider traditional practices and justify them if they can. In other words, an emphasis on clinical freedom asserts the importance of professionalism, and requires the interferer to respect this by demonstrating why it must be narrowed, if it must.

The second benefit that clinical freedom brings to medicine concerns its positive benefit to the doctor–patient relationship. Patients must believe that doctors are making the best judgement they can in the circumstances for the good of patients —

that they are not being influenced by considerations, for example, of race, or of social class. This is another aspect of professionalism. Doctors must always resist becoming agents of the State, or of commercial concerns.

13.3 Independence and individuality

Clinical freedom can easily be ridiculed, as in the pharmaceutical nightmare (13.1.); and one reason for this is that it can fall ambiguously between two different qualities — independence of mind and individuality of mind. Each of these can be thought of as 'having a mind of one's own', but they are essentially different. Individuality is what some people find lacking in a medical life-style; and it is not encouraged by medical education. Its absence can lead to dissatisfaction over the fulfillment of the personal aims (3.3) of the doctor. For example, as we have seen (3.3) there is a criticism sometimes made of medical education that it produces too much uniformity. There are many expressions of this general criticism: that medical students are required to spend too much time on rote learning; that they do not or cannot think for themselves; that there is too much deference to authority and tradition in medicine; that doctors all think alike and dress alike.

Independence of mind is shown in the kind of support or justification a person might offer for a belief, rather than in either the way in which the belief is acquired in the first place or in the content of the belief. For it can be an accident how people acquire their beliefs; they may acquire them through experience, or through books, or from an influential teacher. But, however the belief is acquired, a person shows independence of mind with respect to it in so far as he/she continues to hold the belief on evidence or similar considerations. A person may of course acquire a belief as a result of encountering evidence for it, but equally it may be acquired as a result of parental teaching; nevertheless, independence of mind is shown only if the belief is subsequently based on whatever is the appropriate evidence. Again, students listening to a lecture might all become convinced of the truth of certain propositions. Yet they could all be said to be independent-minded with respect to those beliefs provided they based their beliefs on the argument and the evidence presented (as distinct from the authority of the lecturer), and despite the fact that in the case of each student the content of his belief was the same as that of his fellows. On the other hand, a group (if such exists) of independent-minded, argument-devouring students could not be said to have individuality of mind if they all believed the same; individuality of mind does concern differences in the content of people's beliefs, and is much less concerned with the rational basis of the beliefs. The beliefs of an independent mind are, or purport to be, well-founded; whereas those of an individual mind are or purport to be distinctive, idiosyncratic, or unique.

13.4   Independence of mind

What does independence of mind consist in? The first point here is that we begin to be independent of other people in our thinking to the extent that we base our beliefs on evidence or argument, as distinct from the testimony and authority of others. This sweeping statement must of course be developed and qualified. Different types of evidence are needed in different sorts of situations, and sometimes we ourselves may not be able to state the evidence. For example, if the matter is very technical we may need to rely on the word of experts. But even here we can acquire some ability to assess where expertise is relevant and where it is being abused, as when, say, doctors pronounce on matters outside their competence as doctors. We can also assess someone's title to be regarded as an expert, by asking about qualifications or experience, or consulting others in the same business. So even here our beliefs can be grounded in evidence, but indirectly so.

A second factor which makes us independent-minded is our ability to understand what we claim to have in our minds. For example, supposing a student is told that cimetidine is an H_2 receptor antagonist, and reduces gastric acid secretion. How does the student make this statement 'his own'? He would need to understand concepts like 'H_2 receptor antagonist', and the general significance of acid secretion. Understanding is clearly something we can have more or less of; and to the extent that we have it we are more or less independently minded.

Thirdly, we are independently minded to the extent that we are critical of the evidence or arguments for a belief. We may come to hold that the evidence is insufficient, or of the wrong kind, or that the arguments are weak. Instruction in the critical appraisal of appropriate evidence is indeed one of the characteristics common to any sort of academic discipline. For example a question such as the evidence for the benefits of screening programmes requires critical ability.

Granted then that independence of mind consists in directing our attention to appropriate evidence, in understanding what we claim to believe, and in being critical of these beliefs and the evidence for them, we can now ask two questions: what is the relationship being independently minded and clinical freedom, and what is the relationship between being independently minded and being educated?

Take first the relationship between independence of mind and clinical freedom. The relationship is one of identity in the sense that clinical freedom just is the showing of independence of mind in a clinical contest. Clinical freedom is shown when the doctor's judgement is based on the available scientific knowledge and is tailored to suit the specific conditions and needs of specific patients, within the constraints of law, ethics, and finance. Positive freedom is displayed when the doctor's judgement is developed by knowledge, and negative freedom when that judgement shows awareness of the contemporary constraints. When clinical freedom satisfies these conditions it is identical with independence of mind.

Consider next the relationship between being independently minded and being educated. There seem to be two possibilities. The first is that the connection is causal, that independence of mind 'leads to' or is a factor in creating what we call 'being educated'. In terms of this line of argument the two ideas of independence of mind and educatedness are seen to be independently identifiable, and one is taken to be conducive to the other. But this is not plausible. To see someone as educated is to see that person as being independently minded (in the sense we have outlined); and to see people as independently minded is to see them as (to some extent and in one sense) educated. The relationship between the ideas cannot therefore be causal. We must therefore turn to the second possibility: that the relationship is a logical one. It can be claimed to be part of the definition of educatedness that the educated person should have a mind of his/her own. If this is correct, we can explain the importance we attach to being independently minded, and can justify the pursuit of it. To put it in terms of the processes of education, in helping people to become independently minded we are by the same token helping them to become educated. Hence, there is abundant justification for trying to acquire independence of mind, and for having a mind of one's own, or showing clinical freedom in the medical context.

13.5   Individuality of mind

Let us turn now to the other idea which can be confusingly involved in clinical freedom — individuality of mind. What does individuality of mind consist in?

In the first place, individuality of mind can consist in an unusual direction of interest. The person with the individual mind may know about unusual or less commonly known things, such as Victorian toys, the Grassmarket in the eighteenth century, the science of John of Norfolk, Persian rugs, the songs of troubadours. Secondly, the person of individual mind may have a great depth of knowledge on some subjects. He may concentrate, to the point of obsession, on a few subjects or on just one — in this direction lies the specialist who knows more and more about less and less.

Thirdly, in the case of individuality of mind there are possibilities which do not exist for independence of mind — the former but not the latter can be shown in modes which have nothing to do with evidence or understanding, or indeed are not knowledge-based at all. For example, individuality of mind (but not independence of mind) can be shown in ways of dressing, and indeed in ways of living; a style of life can bear a distinctive signature. The term 'originality' can be used for this third side to individuality, and it is above all in the arts that this kind of individuality is shown, although it is also shown in science or medicine.

Some artists reveal their originality in their ability to make us see the familiar in a new light. For example, Wordsworth and

Coleridge in their *Preface to the Lyrical Ballads* of 1803 said that
in their poetry they intended to remove the film of familiarity
which everyday experience spreads over things. The person
of individual mind can make us appreciate afresh what we
already know. Again, originality can consist in the creation of
new ideas or new styles. For example, Wagner or Schoenberg
might be said to be great innovators in music, Galileo and
Einstein in science, and Kant and Wittgenstein in philosophy.
The interesting point is that whether the creative innovation is
in art or science or philosophy, the result in each case is the
same — the human imagination is enriched, and we can see the
world in fresh ways.

What is the connection between individuality of mind and
clinical freedom, and between individuality and educatedness?

Taking first individuality and clinical freedom, we might be
tempted to say that it represents the pathology of clinical freedom, the eccentric, 'if-it-works-for-you' attitude made fun of in
the pharmaceutical nightmare. This is correct; individuality is
no adequate substitute for a scientifically-based diagnosis (or
independence of mind).

Two qualifications must be made here. The first is that there
is more to treatment than what is known scientifically. We have
already stressed the importance of 'whole-person care; and the
unique nature of each patient. Individuality of mind can come
into its own when medicine is thought of as an art. We shall
return to this point. The second qualification is that eccentricity
can have a place. Sometimes what is called 'the scientific
approach' is simply the repetition of received opinion. It takes
individuality of mind to challenge this; and therefore such individuality does have some bearing on clinical freedom.

Let us turn now to the question of the relationship between
individuality of mind and educatedness. Individuality is certainly not part of the definition of educatedness, for it is neither
necessary nor sufficient for educatedness. It is not necessary,
in that we would not withhold the title of 'educated' from a
person because he/she lacked any or all of the characteristics
mentioned above. For example, students graduate in their
thousands every year who have no unusual direction in their
interests, no particular depth in their knowledge, and no
particular originality; yet it would be doctrinaire to say that

they are not educated, provided they have some independence of mind. It is also not sufficient, in that a person might have an extensive knowledge of something (cricketers of the 1920s), but still not be educated. Indeed, it may well be that some obsessive scholar in a university has an individual mind, but is barely educated. The point here is that being educated, while it does not logically require deep knowledge of anything or knowledge of unusual things, does logically require some breadth of knowledge, and an active curiosity. This is particularly true of medical education. Such qualities are sometimes conspicuously lacking in distinguished specialists, in any discipline.

To maintain that persons with individuality of mind are not for that reason educated is not to say that they are not highly desirable in other ways. Educatedness is only one kind of good, and should be balanced against the obsessive scientist, or the creative artist, or the surgeon who devotes his life to perfecting a difficult technique. These too are good lives. The problem is that while educatedness is logically consistent with individuality of mind, it is psychologically and practically difficult to combine the two, and it is difficult and unusual for a person to have both. Centres of higher education are designed to produce independence of mind, but are poor at producing individuality of mind. The latter claim is perhaps an unfair way of putting the point, since they do not set out to produce individuality of mind. Nevertheless, there is a certain grey uniformity about what comes out of universities. This is certainly true in medicine.

If individuality of mind cannot be justified as being part of the definition of educatedness, how can it be justified, if at all? There are two sorts of justification, one in terms of self-development, and the other in terms of the plural and varied society.

It is from the variety of interests or even the conflict of interests to which individuality of mind gives rise that progress results. Adventures in ideas and in forms of life are necessary if individuals or societies are not to stagnate; and it is those with individuality of mind who are most likely to have such adventures. Applying this point to medical education, we note that while the ideal of producing the all-round, safe practitioner (i.e. one who has independence of mind and is to that extent educated) is no doubt good in many respects, it has three disadvantages, one professional and two personal.

The professional disadvantage is that the cultivation of soundness can be at the expense of sparkle; the eccentric and individual mind can often be the creative one, whether in medical research or in clinical diagnosis. It is perhaps a matter of getting the balance right. The cultivation of breadth of medical knowledge, ability to assess evidence, and the curiosity to update medical knowledge, which are all necessary conditions for the exercise of clinical freedom or medical independence of mind, must remain the major element in medical education. But we have also argued that there must be encouragement, and space, in the curriculum to cultivate individuality. This too has a contribution to make to clinical freedom.

It has even more of a contribution to make to the personal fulfillment of the doctor in his professional work. The gifts and skills of doctors are various, and if medicine is to progress and doctors are to feel that their personal aims are fulfilled in medicine there must be scope and encouragement for experiments and innovations in practice. That encouragement should begin in the undergraduate curriculum. Finally, the criticism often made of doctors, that they are a homogeneous, inward-looking, and professionally self-absorbed group, can also be answered if scope is left in the curriculum for an interest in something other than medicine.

13.6   Conclusions

1. 'Clinical freedom' is central to the make-up of a doctor, and its cultivation is part of the hidden agenda of medical education.

2. It can seem educationally defensible because 'having a mind of one's own' is often thought to be identical with being educated, and clinical freedom is having a mind of one's own in a clinical context.

3. But 'having a mind of one's own' is ambiguous as between 'independence of mind' and 'individuality of mind'. Clinical freedom properly understood is a medical expression of independence of mind, and is therefore part of educatedness. But individuality of mind also has something to contribute to clinical freedom, and to the fulfillment of the personal aims of a doctor in public and private life.

Bibliography

Sheldon B. (1978). Theory and practice in social work: a re-examination of a tenuous relationship. *The British Journal of Social Work*, 8(1), 6–7. (Quoted with permission.)

Straughan, R. and Wilson, J. (eds) (1987). *Philosophers on education.* Macmillan, London.

14 Strategies for change

14.1 Institutional inertia

It is one thing to propose sensible and useful reforms to medical education; it is quite another to get them adopted. There is a gap between theory and practice, which exists even when the proposed theory is widely acknowledged to be a good one, and the current practice a bad one. One explanation for this gap is institutional inertia.

Institutional inertia is not always a bad thing. It is one aspect of those traditional practices of medical schools which, as we have already stated, encapsulate much that is distinctive and valuable about the education they provide. Inertia is the opposite of agitation; and a university whose teachers and curriculum were in a constant state of flux would be unable to furnish or enforce standards. Nevertheless, there are times when inertia must be overcome, and the complex system of interlocking structures, checks, and balances must be forced into motion.

This chapter attempts to identify strategies by which constructive change may be encouraged. Different institutions have different strengths, problems, and structures, and are staffed and attended by miscellaneous assorted personalities: therefore any suggestions are necessarily general in nature. None the less, some useful clarification is possible.

This discussion of means and ends may seem to have overtones of Machiavelli's advice in *The prince* concerning the various techniques of seizing and maintaining power (at any cost) — but this would be misleading. Even if it were possible to have one's educational enemies put to the sword, their offices sown with salt, and compliant puppets installed in their places — this would still result in a situation entirely inimical to good education. ... It is vital that educational change is motivated by positive goals, and occurs with the consent (if not the approval!) of teachers and students.

14.2 Attitudes

As a preliminary to change there must be an atmosphere of dissatisfaction with the status quo combined with a perception of the possibility of constructive reform. If there is no such perception, then both the possibility and desirability of change are greatly diminished. Such a mood may be generated by articles and books (such as this one perhaps), by conversation, by grassroots (i.e. student) or top-down (managerial) initiatives. Given such an environment, there will initially tend to be a profusion of ideas and notions, some well-formed and some half-baked (this situation was characteristic of the educational debate of the late 1960s and early 1970s). At first it is a matter of 'let a thousand flowers bloom'; none the less, before too long good horticultural practice dictates the need for weeding, so that the more deserving plants are given the chance to thrive.

The development of a mood for change is largely the development of a change in attitudes. Within an educational institution such as a medical school or university it might be expected that attitudes to educational practice would be a subject of intense and open-minded debate. This is by no means the case, and it is possible for staff and students to cruise along for many years without fully confronting the possibility that their attitudes may be mistaken. How, then, can attitudes be changed?

An attitude is not something which exists in isolation. Individual attitudes are part of whole networks which are more or less closely linked to make up part of what we call a personality. Furthermore, attitudes are not only linked horizontally with others, but have a variable depth of conviction — some are held more strongly than others. Attitudes, then, are stable to the extent that they are embedded in networks, yet open to change in that when one is altered this may have an effect on many others. Of course people are not always consistent in terms of attitudes — attitudes may contradict each other, or be contradicted by behaviour. This can lead to cognitive imbalance or dissonance between attitudes: for example, a schoolboy may believe that smoking is dirty and dangerous, and yet admire a football hero who smokes, or a lecturer may accept a salary to teach and examine a syllabus which she believes is fundamentally misguided. The contradiction inherent in such situations renders the system unstable, and either one or the other attitude or behaviour is liable to change so as to bring the whole complex into a consistent relationship.

The reformer can thus work from agreed principles (for example, 'We should teach students to think for themselves') to highlight contradictory practice (for example, students are lectured at from nine-to-five, with no opportunity for feedback) and amplify the cognitive dissonance, while recognizing that the paradox can be resolved in more than one direction, and also that people are remarkably good at just living with paradox.

14.3   Forms of communication

One major question concerns the form of communication designed to encourage educational change. This is particularly important in the light of a phenomenon called 'selective exposure'. Generally speaking, people will 'expose' themselves only to information which is consonant with their attitudes, so that a Conservative voter might be expected to read the *Daily Telegraph* but to avoid Labour party political broadcasts. Exceptions to this hypothesis occur either when the attitudes are undogmatically held, or else when the attitudes are so strongly held that the person is confident of defeating any challenge to their value-system.

Nevertheless, attitudes do change in response to information, and we are drawn to consider how doctors and other medical teachers come into contact with new information. Broadly speaking there are two ways; spoken and written. Of course doctors as citizens are exposed to the full range of media coverage, which includes health and educational issues; but we have argued that one distinguishing feature of doctors is their high level of professionalization, one feature of which is that doctors are influenced by their colleagues more than by anyone else. And doctors communicate with each other mostly by talking and through the professional journals.

Here we again come across one major problem: 'the medical education ghetto'. The fact is that most of the discussion of medical education is 'preaching to the converted', and once somebody is an attender at education conferences, or a reader of *Medical Teacher*, or a buyer of books such as this one they have already agreed to the need for change, and are just wrangling over details. The problem involves those people who have done none of these things and are never likely to do so.

We must therefore have talkers and writers about medical education who are impressive to and respected by those uninterested in medical education: we need to have the prestigious, the admirable, and the entertaining on our side. And they must extend their activities, as much as possible, beyond the academic rigours of the medical education ghetto and into the hurly-burly, pragmatic world of generally attended lectures, face-to-face talks with a diversity of practising doctors and academics, and the high-circulation, high-impact medical journals and magazines. Out of the ivory tower and into the surgery!

14.4　Institutional barriers

Quite aside from, and perhaps in complete contrast to, the attitudes of individual staff taken one at a time, we have the 'group dynamic' of an institution and its subdivisions. Any change to educational practice will thus come up against the existing power structures, which, in the case of British universities, are usually departments (or their equivalent). Hence the medical curriculum is often divided into semi-autonomous disciplines, each of which is responsible for teaching and scholarship. This system has much to recommend it, not least in terms of simplicity. Nevertheless, it is open to question whether a collection of such departments, each working to safeguard its own vested interests, can produce a sensible curriculum. Much depends upon the relative status and force of personality associated with heads of departments.

On the other hand, there is a contemporary trend to separate the organization of teaching and research, so that teaching is organized on the basis of courses, while research teams are flexible *ad hoc* formations, frequently of an interdisciplinary nature. Such a system may indeed be more open to change; but there are other power structures to contend with, and the difficulties are better regarded as being displaced rather than dissolved.

The possibility of change always brings with it a threat to established organizational (and individual) control, status, and perhaps freedom. It is also a challenge to the expertise of existing staff; there is a criticism of their present work which is implicit in the very idea that change is needed. When departments typically exert the major control over appointments and promotions, it may be that the requirement for 'supra-departmental' forms of activity in educational reform may be regarded as somewhat treacherous to the discipline or the department (just as research activity outside the departmental boundaries is often frowned upon). For these and other reasons, an automatic scepticism and resistance is likely to be the initial reaction to discussion concerning the need for change — whatever the content of the changes proposed.

One strategy is to sidestep institutional barriers by side-stepping the educational institution itself, and forming a 'pressure group'. Thus we have multi-disciplinary organizations such as the Association for the study of Medical Education. Alternatively there are broader-based organizations which take an interest in medical education, such as the King's Fund or, more famously, the General Medical Council. All of these organizations have made substantial contributions to medical education; and we have argued above that the GMC might engage in a bit more sabre-rattling to ensure that its recommendations are taken seriously.

Nevertheless, the advantage of detachment from institutional pressures is also a disadvantage in the sense that 'pressure group' pronouncements are easily ignored by institutions as being too idealistic, too generalized, or in some other way inappropriate for any specific medical school or university. The most difficult task involves building bridges between 'pressure groups' and the organizations which it is hoped will implement their recommendations.

14.5   Resource implications

Resources include money, time, and space/facilities. Reformers should not underestimate the requirement for these in implementing any new idea. The need for money and adequate physical means are obvious; but the time spent discussing and planning educational changes is equally important. Medical schools are, of course, primarily concerned with teaching and research in a clinical setting, and hours of committee wrangling must accept a relatively low priority. Participants must be convinced that the goals are worthwhile, and that an initial investment of time and energy will be amply repaid in the longer run. And it is notoriously difficult to obtain agreement on the results of educational change: for example, the endless controversy over contradictory evidence on whether children's reading 'standards' are rising, falling, or staying the same. Notwithstanding, although financial resources are likely to remain at present levels — or even decline — people are often remarkably generous with their effort when they perceive that they are working towards valuable objectives.

14.6 Personal incentives

In so far as medical educators are affected by sticks and carrots, which is probably as much as most people, it is noticeable that the priority afforded to educational endeavour comes well below clinical excellence and research performance. Furthermore, while good teaching ability within the current framework may attract favourable notice to a member of staff, an interest in broader educational issues is looked upon with some disapproval, as probable evidence of a second-rate mind! Good teaching is taken to mean good lecturing or tutoring, and as such to be divorced from the organization and its essential aims; 'education(al)ist' is a term of abuse in some medical (and university) circles — more or less the semantic equivalent of soft-boiled, trendy, lefty, and lazy. Studying the forms (as opposed to the content) of teaching and learning remains of dubious value, even to those whose job is education. Finally, publications and prestige in terms of educational topics would probably 'not count' when it came to assessing staff achievement: medical education is not considered a part of medicine, and time spent on the subject is seen as time wasted.

It is a truism of managerial theory (although one which is usually ignored) that for effective change to become established in 'expert' activities such as clinical medicine or teaching the participants must enjoy a sense of 'ownership' of the process.

There is thus no place in medical education for the unilateral imposition of detailed blueprints; plans must be subjected to a process of broad consultation and consensus-building, and be responsive both to their influence and also to the influence of those who will implement them, which will vary from one situation to another. This recommendation is in line with our commitment to maintain individual traditions and excellences in medical education — building upon local strengths.

Furthermore, if creative involvement is required, then plans cannot be too specific, but must leave space for initiative. This implies that plans must have at least four levels of increasing specificity: a set of general principles coming down from 'on high' (from, for example, the GMC) following consultation; the selection from such principles those that are appropriate for each institution, and a parcelling-out of these among departments (or their equivalents); departmental modifications in the light of staff and facilities; and finally the creative involvement of individual teachers to take account of their own abilities and the best interests of the students. Such good educational practice is highly demanding of individual effort, and is deserving of institutional recognition through the normal channels (honourable mention, increments, promotions, titles, prizes, or whatever).

14.7   Radical or conservative change?

It is our contention that many of the medical reformers of the 1970s were 'too radical', which is why they failed. This criticism takes two forms, the pragmatic and the idealistic.

The pragmatic criticism is that when a reform is too radical it becomes impossible. What happens is that a too-radical measure is irrational in terms of the existing structure: before anything can change everything must change; because everything cannot change, nothing will change. The stakes are too high, the process is just too expensive and too risky. The exception is when a new institution is built from the ground up, with new staff appointed on a new understanding of their role. This has been the case in the USA (most famously in Case Western Reserve), in Europe (for example, at Maastricht), and in other countries — but not in Britain.

In a sense the British are victims of their own success. Medical education here is too good, contains too much of value, for us even to want to tear it all down and start afresh. So, whatever the pragmatic possibilities, even on purely idealistic grounds we do not want to change everything, because we do not want to throw the baby out with the bathwater.

This leads on to the desirability of piecemeal change, of gradualism, so that the innovative is tested before it gains acceptance, and the best of established practice is conserved. Throughout this book we have tried to present our proposals in the form of discrete measures which can each be introduced individually while leaving the rest of the system intact. Such a method fits neatly into the currently fashionable idea of modular organization for degree courses: new ideas can be introduced as modules, or part-modules.

It is important to remember that, no matter how reasonable an educational innovation might seem, its full implications can never be predicted — the possible range of interactions are just too complex. In this respect it is like any other human activity — politics, health care, or whatever — and should follow a pattern of hypothesis, experiment (or pilot study), and evaluation before being adopted firmly. This modest and scientific approach is likely to win the support even of those who are sceptical of reform. When it is clear that a proposal is not all or nothing, never or for ever, but is subject to appraisal and rejection if it has failed to achieve its objectives, then opponents may be prepared to try it and see. To work, this scientific approach must have predetermined goals and a pre-established trial period; but the acceptance of the proposal must not be predetermined, but instead must be subject to a decision on its success or failure according to agreed criteria.

14.8 Why bother?

If constructive change is so complex and hard to manage, why bother with it? Especially as there is widespread cynicism about whether education has any significant effect at all! Perhaps character is fixed while we are still at school; perhaps we forget everything we have ever been taught; perhaps institutional pressures (organization, examination syllabuses, or whatever) will always sabotage high educational ideals? Why not just accept things as they are, and try to teach and work as well as possible within the existing system? There are many answers; but here are some of those which seem most convincing to us.

The first is that *laissez faire* is a recipe for decline. Medical practice changes, students change, and education will not stay the same: it will become worse. The price of excellence is eternal vigilance: if we stop trying to improve we will start to deteriorate.

The second answer is the innate tendency of institutions to become hermetically sealed from the rest of the world — 'institutional drift' — and to become pedantic and irrelevant, concerned only with petty internal squabbles and triumphs. This is particularly problematic in the highly professional world of medicine, where external criticism is so easily ignored. Yet it is of particular importance in medicine that we think *who* and *how* we are educating, because the end-result may be practising on us for forty years.

And the third answer concerns human enjoyment. We believe that medical education could be much more enjoyable for all concerned. It is scandalous that preclinical students are force-fed facts for seven hours a day, that a consultant's teaching ward-round — the major method of clinical teaching — can be accurately encapsulated as 'shifting dullness', that the 'best years' of a young doctor's life may be spent sitting (and re-sitting) postgraduate exams of unknown validity and doubtful utility ... It seems to us that the onus of proof lies most upon those who contend that such tedious practices are *essential* to good medicine, rather than upon those who propose change. Even if educational reform did nothing more than make life more interesting and enjoyable it would be worth doing. After all, anything which serves to reinforce and refresh the human spirit must be a good thing — especially in medicine.

Bibliography

Mennin, S. P. and Kaufman, A. (1989). The change process and medical education. *Medical Teacher*, **11**, 1–9.

Martenson, D. (1989). Educational development in an established medical school: facilitating and impeding factors in change at the Korlinska Institute. *Medical Teacher*, **11**, 9–25.

Index